Pulmonary Vascular Disease

Editor

JEFFREY P. KANNE

RADIOLOGIC CLINICS OF NORTH AMERICA

www.radiologic.theclinics.com

Consulting Editor
FRANK H. MILLER

March 2025 • Volume 63 • Number 2

ELSEVIER

1600 John F. Kennedy Boulevard • Suite 1800 • Philadelphia, Pennsylvania, 19103-2899

http://www.theclinics.com

RADIOLOGIC CLINICS OF NORTH AMERICA Volume 63, Number 2
March 2025 ISSN 0033-8389, ISBN 13: 978-0-443-29482-2

Editor: John Vassallo (j.vassallo@elsevier.com)
Developmental Editor: Malvika Shah

© **2025 Elsevier Inc. All rights are reserved, including those for text and data mining, AI training, and similar technologies.**

This periodical and the individual contributions contained in it are protected under copyright by Elsevier, and the following terms and conditions apply to their use:

Photocopying
Single photocopies of single articles may be made for personal use as allowed by national copyright laws. Permission of the Publisher and payment of a fee is required for all other photocopying, including multiple or systematic copying, copying for advertising or promotional purposes, resale, and all forms of document delivery. Special rates are available for educational institutions that wish to make photocopies for non-profit educational classroom use. For information on how to seek permission visit www.elsevier.com/permissions or call: (+44) 1865 843830 (UK)/(+1) 215 239 3804 (USA).

Derivative Works
Subscribers may reproduce tables of contents or prepare lists of articles including abstracts for internal circulation within their institutions. Permission of the Publisher is required for resale or distribution outside the institution. Permission of the Publisher is required for all other derivative works, including compilations and translations (please consult www.elsevier.com/permissions).

Electronic Storage or Usage
Permission of the Publisher is required to store or use electronically any material contained in this periodical, including any article or part of an article (please consult www.elsevier.com/permissions). Except as outlined above, no part of this publication may be reproduced, stored in a retrieval system or transmitted in any form or by any means, electronic, mechanical, photocopying, recording or otherwise, without prior written permission of the Publisher.

Notice
No responsibility is assumed by the Publisher for any injury and/or damage to persons or property as a matter of products liability, negligence or otherwise, or from any use or operation of any methods, products, instructions or ideas contained in the material herein. Because of rapid advances in the medical sciences, in particular, independent verification of diagnoses and drug dosages should be made.

Although all advertising material is expected to conform to ethical (medical) standards, inclusion in this publication does not constitute a guarantee or endorsement of the quality or value of such product or of the claims made of it by its manufacturer.

Radiologic Clinics of North America (ISSN 0033-8389) is published bimonthly by Elsevier Inc., 360 Park Avenue South, New York, NY 10010-1710. Months of issue are January, March, May, July, September, and November. Periodicals postage paid at New York, NY and additional mailing offices. Subscription prices are USD 566 per year for US individuals, USD 100 per year for US students and residents, USD 649 per year for Canadian individuals, USD 761 per year for international individuals, USD 100 per year for Canadian students/residents, and USD 315 per year for international students/residents. For institutional access pricing please contact Customer Service via the contact information below. To receive student and resident rate, orders must be accompanied by name of affiliated institution, date of term and the signature of program/residency coordinatior on institution letterhead. Orders will be billed at individual rate until proof of status is received. Foreign air speed delivery is included in all *Clinics* subscription prices. All prices are subject to change without notice. Orders, claims, and journal inquiries: Please visit our Support Hub page https://service.elsevier.com for assistance.

Reprints. For copies of 100 or more of articles in this publication, please contact the Commercial Reprints Department, Elsevier Inc., 360 Park Avenue South, New York, New York 10010-1710. Tel.: +1-212-633-3874; Fax: +1-212-633-3820; E-mail: reprints@elsevier.com.

Radiologic Clinics of North America also published in Greek Paschalidis Medical Publications, Athens, Greece.

Radiologic Clinics of North America is covered in MEDLINE/PubMed (Index Medicus), EMBASE/Excerpta Medica, Current Contents/Life Sciences, Current Contents/Clinical Medicine, RSNA Index to Imaging Literature, BIOSIS, Science Citation Index, and ISI/BIOMED.

Printed in the United States of America.

Pulmonary Vascular Disease

Contributors

CONSULTING EDITOR

FRANK H. MILLER, MD, FACR
Lee F. Rogers, MD, Professor of Medical Education; Chief, Body Imaging Section; Medical Director, MRI; Professor, Department of Radiology, Northwestern Memorial Hospital, Northwestern University, Feinberg School of Medicine, Chicago, Illinois

EDITOR

JEFFREY P. KANNE, MD
Professor (CHS) and Chief of Thoracic Imaging, Department of Radiology, University of Wisconsin School of Medicine and Public Health, Madison, Wisconsin

AUTHORS

HANNAH AHN, MD
Cardiothoracic Radiologist, Department of Radiology and Biomedical Imaging, University of California San Francisco, San Francisco, California

BRADLEY D. ALLEN, MD
Assistant Professor, Department of Radiology, Northwestern University Feinberg School of Medicine, Chicago, Illinois

KIRAN BATRA, MD
Associate Professor, Cardiothoracic Imaging, Departments of Radiology and Internal Medicine, University of Texas Southwestern Medical Center, Dallas, Texas

DONALD BENSON, MD, PhD
Assistant Professor, Cardiopulmonary Imaging Section, Department of Radiology, University of Alabama at Birmingham, Birmingham, Alabama

CATHERINE BODNAR, MD
Resident, Department of Pathology and Laboratory Medicine, University of Wisconsin, Madison, Wisconsin

JONATHAN H. CHUNG, MD
Professor, Department of Radiology, University of California San Diego, La Jolla, California

MARGARITA CONSING-GANGELHOFF, MD
Resident, Department of Pathology and Laboratory Medicine, University of Wisconsin, Madison, Wisconsin

ERIC CROTTY, MD
Assistant Professor, Department of Radiology, Cincinnati Children's Hospital Medical Center, Cincinnati, Ohio

SAYEDOMID EBRAHIMZADEH, MD
Clinical Instructor, Department of Radiology and Biomedical Imaging, University of California San Francisco, San Francisco, California

JOANNA G. ESCALON, MD
Assistant Professor, Division of Cardiothoracic Imaging, Department of Radiology, New York-Presbyterian Hospital, Weill Cornell Medical Center, New York, New York

Contributors

KARA N. GOSS, MD
Associate Professor, Departments of Medicine and Pediatrics, UT Southwestern Medical Center, Dallas, Texas

MEGAN GRIFFITHS, MD
Assistant Professor, Department of Pediatrics, UT Southwestern Medical Center, Dallas, Texas

R. PAUL GUILLERMAN, MD
Professor, Department of Radiology, Cincinnati Children's Hospital Medical Center, Cincinnati, Ohio

LEWIS D. HAHN, MD
Associate Professor, Department of Radiology, University of California San Diego, La Jolla, California

BRANDON R. JAKUBOWSKI, MD
Assistant Professor, Department of Medicine, UT Southwestern Medical Center, Dallas, Texas

JEFFREY P. KANNE, MD
Professor (CHS), Department of Radiology, University of Wisconsin, Madison, Wisconsin

FERNANDO U. KAY, MD, PhD
Associate Professor, Cardiothoracic Imaging, Department of Radiology, University of Texas Southwestern Medical Center, Dallas, Texas

GRACE LAIDLAW, MD, MS
Assistant Professor, Section of Interventional Radiology, Department of Radiology, University of Washington, Seattle, Washington

LARRY A. LATSON Jr, MD, MS
Assistant Professor, Division of Cardiothoracic Imaging, Department of Radiology, New York-Presbyterian Hospital, Weill Cornell Medical Center, New York, New York

CHRISTOPHER LEE, MD
Assistant Professor, Department of Radiology and Biomedical Imaging, University of California San Francisco, San Francisco, California

JONATHAN LIU, MD, MS
Assistant Professor, Department of Radiology and Biomedical Imaging, University of California San Francisco, San Francisco, California

HUGH McGREGOR, MD
Associate Professor, Section of Interventional Radiology, Department of Radiology, University of Washington, Seattle, Washington

RONALD M. PESHOCK, MD
Professor and Vice Chair Information Technology for Radiology, Cardiothoracic, Division Radiology, Departments of Radiology and Internal Medicine, University of Texas Southwestern Medical Center, Dallas, Texas

ALEXANDER PHAN, MD
Assistant Professor, Division of Cardiothoracic Imaging, Department of Radiology, New York-Presbyterian Hospital, Weill Cornell Medical Center, New York, New York

ANDREW SCHAPIRO, MD
Assistant Professor, Department of Radiology, Cincinnati Children's Hospital Medical Center, Cincinnati, Ohio

JEFREE J. SCHULTE, MD
Assistant Professor, Department of Pathology and Laboratory Medicine, University of Wisconsin, Madison, Wisconsin

MARK SHAROBIM, MD
Resident, Department of Pathology and Laboratory Medicine, University of Wisconsin, Madison, Wisconsin

ROBERT C. SIBLEY, MD
Assistant Professor, Nuclear Medicine, Cardiothoracic Imaging, Department of Radiology, University of Texas Southwestern Medical Center, Dallas, Texas

SHRAVAN SRIDHAR, MD, MS
Assistant Professor, Department of Radiology and Biomedical Imaging, University of California San Francisco, San Francisco, California

AKI TANIMOTO, MD
Assistant Professor, Department of Radiology, Cincinnati Children's Hospital Medical Center, Cincinnati, Ohio

TUGCE AGIRLAR TRABZONLU, MD
Assistant Professor, Department of Radiology, Northwestern University Feinberg School of Medicine, Chicago, Illinois

KARIM VALJI, MD
Professor, Section of Interventional Radiology, Department of Radiology, University of Washington, Seattle, Washington

DANIEL VARGAS, MD
Associate Professor, Division of Cardiopulmonary Imaging, Department of Radiology, University of Colorado School of Medicine, Aurora, Colorado

Contents

Preface: Imaging of Pulmonary Vascular Disease, xv

Jeffrey P. Kanne

Pathology of Pulmonary Vascular Disease with Radiologic Correlation 179

Margarita Consing-Gangelhoff, Mark Sharobim, Catherine Bodnar, Jeffrey P. Kanne, and Jefree J. Schulte

> Pulmonary hypertensive changes are commonly seen by the surgical pathologist, but the majority represents secondary changes due to some process extrinsic to the lung. Some primary, or idiopathic, vascular diseases result in unique pathologic changes including the plexiform lesion and venous hypertensive changes. Thromboembolic disease also shows unique pathologic features. Diffuse alveolar hemorrhage, vasculitis, and capillaritis often overlap, but may represent separate, distinct pathologic processes. Lastly, alveolar capillary dysplasia with misalignment of pulmonary veins, as well as chronic lung allograft vasculopathy, present as unique pathologies in the neonate and posttransplant recipient, respectively.

Imaging Approach to Pulmonary Hypertension 193

Shravan Sridhar, Sayedomid Ebrahimzadeh, Hannah Ahn, Christopher Lee, and Jonathan Liu

> Pulmonary hypertension is a rare but important clinical problem that presents a sometimes challenging diagnostic dilemma. The diagnosis of pulmonary hypertension relies on a combination of clinical testing and radiologic imaging, with chest computed tomography (CT) often serving as the primary imaging modality for comprehensive evaluation of the chest. Chest CT can be used to evaluate for causes of pulmonary hypertension including chronic lung disease, pulmonary artery obstruction, and congenital heart disease. Recognizing common appearances of these conditions will enable expedient diagnosis.

Imaging of Acute Pulmonary Embolism: An Update 207

Kiran Batra, Fernando U. Kay, Robert C. Sibley, and Ronald M. Peshock

> Imaging is essential in the evaluation and management of acute pulmonary embolism. Advances in multi-energy CT including dual-energy CT and photon-counting CT have allowed faster scans with lower radiation dose and optimal quality. Artificial intelligence has a potential role in triaging potentially positive examinations and could serve as a second reader.

Imaging of Chronic Thromboembolic Pulmonary Hypertension 223

Lewis D. Hahn and Jonathan H. Chung

> Chronic thromboembolic pulmonary hypertension (CTEPH) is pulmonary hypertension secondary to chronic obstruction of pulmonary arteries by organized thromboemboli. Echocardiography and Echocardiography and ventilation/perfusion (V/Q) scan are the initial screening examinations for CTEPH; the diagnosis is often missed on computed tomography (CT). Imaging findings of chronic thromboembolic pulmonary disease overlap with those of acute pulmonary embolism, and radiologists should evaluate for the presence of concurrent chronic disease in all cases of

acute pulmonary embolism detected on CT pulmonary angiography. Conditions that can mimic CTEPH include in situ thrombus, vasculitis, pulmonary artery sarcoma, and fibrosing mediastinitis.

Imaging of Pulmonary Vasculitis 235
Donald Benson

This review will describe various disease processes resulting in pulmonary vasculitis. The clinical and imaging findings in these diseases often overlap with diffuse alveolar hemorrhage secondary to pulmonary capillaritis, a common manifestation in many of these diseases. A multidisciplinary approach is important for the correct diagnosis of these diseases, and this review will highlight the important imaging findings that radiologists need to be aware of to aid in this diagnostic process.

Congenital Pulmonary Vascular Anomalies and Disease 251
Alexander Phan, Larry A. Latson Jr, Daniel Vargas, and Joanna G. Escalon

Congenital pulmonary vascular disease is a daunting and diverse topic spanning both pulmonary arterial and venous anomalies. Given advancements in treatment, patients with congenital anomalies have longer life expectancies into adulthood and practicing radiologists are bound to come across these patients during their daily practice. Additionally, many anomalies are discovered incidentally on imaging, yet may still have implications for patient care. This article provides an overview of entities most likely encountered in adulthood, highlighting key pre-operative and post-operative imaging features and relevant clinical considerations.

Neonatal and Pediatric Pulmonary Vascular Disease 265
Aki Tanimoto, R. Paul Guillerman, Eric Crotty, and Andrew Schapiro

Pediatric patients are affected by a wide variety of pulmonary vascular diseases ranging from congenital anomalies diagnosed at birth to acquired diseases that present later in childhood and into adolescence. While some pulmonary vascular diseases present similarly to those seen in adults, other forms are unique to children. Knowledge of the characteristic imaging features of these diseases is essential to facilitate prompt diagnosis and guide clinical management.

Role of Cardiovascular MR Imaging and MR Angiography in Patients with Pulmonary Vascular Disease 279
Tugce Agirlar Trabzonlu and Bradley D. Allen

 Video content accompanies this article at http://www.radiologic.theclinics.com.

Cardiac MR imaging and pulmonary MR angiography (MRA) are important clinical tools for the assessment of pulmonary vascular diseases. There are evolving non-contrast and contrast-enhanced techniques to evaluate pulmonary vasculature. Pulmonary MRA is a feasible imaging alternative to CTA in pulmonary embolism detection. Perfusion MR imaging and cardiac MR imaging help diagnose and monitor the treatment response of chronic thromboembolic pulmonary hypertension. Cardiac MR imaging is pivotal in assessing the potential underlying etiology and impact of pulmonary hypertension on the heart. Multiphasic acquisitions and dynamic phase imaging are unique to pulmonary MRA, which aid in diagnosing many pulmonary vascular diseases, including shunts and masses.

Pulmonary Vascular Interventions 293

Grace Laidlaw, Hugh McGregor, and Karim Valji

Endovascular intervention is a safe, effective treatment modality in the management of diverse pulmonary vascular pathologies, including acute or chronic thromboembolic disease, pulmonary arteriovenous malformations (pAVMs), pulmonary artery or bronchial artery hemorrhage, and foreign body retrieval. This article reviews indications, contraindications, techniques, and outcomes in endovascular management of common pulmonary vascular pathologies, with the goal of improving operator familiarity and facility with these procedures.

The Role of Imaging in Pulmonary Vascular Disease: The Clinician's Perspective 305

Brandon R. Jakubowski, Megan Griffiths, and Kara N. Goss

Pulmonary vascular diseases, particularly when accompanied by pulmonary hypertension, are complex disorders often requiring multimodal imaging for diagnosis and monitoring. Echocardiography is the primary screening tool for pulmonary hypertension, while cardiac MR imaging (CMR) is used for more detailed characterization and risk stratification in right ventricular failure. Chest computed tomography (CT) is used to detect vascular anomalies and parenchymal lung diseases. While CT angiography is preferred for the detection of acute pulmonary embolus, dual-energy CT, single photon emission CT, and ventilation/perfusion scintigraphy are recommended for the detection of chronic thromboembolic disease. Application of these modalities will be reviewed here.

PROGRAM OBJECTIVE
The objective of the *Radiologic Clinics of North America* is to keep practicing radiologists and radiology residents up to date with current clinical practice in radiology by providing timely articles reviewing the state of the art in patient care.

TARGET AUDIENCE
Practicing radiologists, radiology residents, and other healthcare professionals who provide patient care utilizing radiologic findings.

LEARNING OBJECTIVES
Upon completion of this activity, participants will be able to:
1. Describe the importance of a multidisciplinary approach for correctly diagnosing pulmonary vasculitis.
2. Discuss the primary imaging modality for pulmonary hypertension.
3. Recognize a thorough understanding of the indications, contraindications, evidence for, and technical approaches to pulmonary vascular interventions are key to effective endovascular management.

ACCREDITATION
The Elsevier Office of Continuing Medical Education (EOCME) is accredited by the Accreditation Council for Continuing Medical Education (ACCME) to provide continuing medical education for physicians.

The EOCME designates this journal-based CME activity for a maximum of 10 *AMA PRA Category 1 Credit*(s)™. Physicians should claim only the credit commensurate with the extent of their participation in the activity.

All other healthcare professionals requesting continuing education credit for this enduring material will be issued a certificate of participation.

DISCLOSURE OF RELEVANT FINANCIAL RELATIONSHIPS
The EOCME assesses conflict of interest with its instructors, faculty, planners, and other individuals who are in a position to control the content of CME activities. All relevant conflicts of interest that are identified are thoroughly vetted by EOCME for fair balance, scientific objectivity, and patient care recommendations. EOCME is committed to providing its learners with CME activities that promote improvements or quality in healthcare and not a specific proprietary business or a commercial interest.

The authors and editors listed below have identified no financial relationships or relationships to products or devices they have with ineligible companies related to the content of this CME activity:
Hannah Ahn, MD; Bradley David Allen, MD; Kiran Batra, MD; Donald Benson, MD; Catherine Bodnar, MD; Jonathan H. Chung, MD; Margarita Consing-Gangelhoff, MD; Eric Crotty, MD; Sayedomid Ebrahimzadeh, MD; Joanna G. Escalon, MD; Kara N. Goss, MD; Megan Griffiths, MD; R. Paul Guillerman, MD; Lewis D. Hahn, MD; Brandon R. Jakubowski, MD; Jeffrey P. Kanne, MD; Fernando U. Kay, MD, PhD; Grace Laidlaw, MD, MS; Larry Latson, MD; Christopher Lee, MD; Jonathan Liu, MD, MS; Hugh McGregor, MD; Alexander Phan, MD; Andrew Schapiro, MD; Jefree J. Schulte, MD; Mark Sharobim, MD; Robert C. Sibley, MD; Shravan Sridhar, MD, MS; Aki Tanimoto, MD; Tugce Agirlar Trabzonlu, MD; Karim Valji, MD; Daniel Vargas, MD

The authors and editors listed below have identified financial relationships or relationships to products or devices they have with ineligible companies related to the content of this CME activity:
Ronald M. Peshock, MD: *Researcher*: Aidoc, Siemens

The planning committee and staff listed below have identified no financial relationships or relationships to products or devices they have with ineligible companies related to the content of this CME activity:
Kothainayaki Kulanthaivelu; Michelle Littlejohn; Patrick J. Manley; Malvika Shah; John Vassallo

UNAPPROVED/OFF-LABEL USE DISCLOSURE
The EOCME requires CME faculty to disclose to the participants:
1. When products or procedures being discussed are off-label, unlabelled, experimental, and/or investigational (not US Food and Drug Administration [FDA] approved); and
2. Any limitations on the information presented, such as data that are preliminary or that represent ongoing research, interim analyses, and/or unsupported opinions. Faculty may discuss information about pharmaceutical agents that is outside of FDA-approved labelling. This information is intended solely for CME and is not intended to promote off-label use of these medications. If you have any questions, contact the medical affairs department of the manufacturer for the most recent prescribing information.

TO ENROLL
To enroll in the *Radiologic Clinics of North America* Continuing Medical Education program, call customer service at 1-800-654-2452 or sign up online at http://www.theclinics.com/home/cme. The CME program is available to subscribers for an additional annual fee of USD 340.00.

METHOD OF PARTICIPATION
In order to claim credit, participants must complete the following:
1. Complete enrolment as indicated above.
2. Read the activity.
3. Complete the CME Test and Evaluation. Participants must achieve a score of 70% on the test. All CME Tests and Evaluations must be completed online.

CME INQUIRIES/SPECIAL NEEDS
For all CME inquiries or special needs, please contact elsevierCME@elsevier.com.

RADIOLOGIC CLINICS OF NORTH AMERICA

FORTHCOMING ISSUES

May 2025
Imaging of the Small Bowel and Colon
Shannon P. Sheedy and Kevin J. Chang, *Editors*

July 2025
Pearls and Pitfalls in Thoracic Disease Imaging
Mylene T. Truong and Girish S. Shroff, *Editors*

September 2025
Advances in Pediatric Imaging
Edward Y. Lee, *Editor*

RECENT ISSUES

January 2025
Ultrasound
Mark E. Lockhart, *Editor*

November 2024
Current Controversies in Diagnostic and Interventional Radiology
Douglas S. Katz and John J. Hines Jr, *Editors*

September 2024
Imaging in Rheumatology
Alberto Bazzocchi and Giuseppe Guglielmi, *Editors*

SERIES OF RELATED INTEREST

Advances in Clinical Radiology
Available at: https://www.advancesinclinicalradiology.com/
Magnetic Resonance Imaging Clinics
Available at: https://www.mri.theclinics.com/
Neuroimaging Clinics
Available at: www.neuroimaging.theclinics.com
PET Clinics
Available at: www.pet.theclinics.com

THE CLINICS ARE AVAILABLE ONLINE!
Access your subscription at:
www.theclinics.com

Preface
Imaging of Pulmonary Vascular Disease

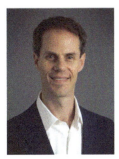

Jeffrey P. Kanne, MD
Editor

Pulmonary vascular disease is often overlooked as a cause of patients presenting with respiratory signs and symptoms. However, nearly every imaging examination of the chest performed shows in some way the state of the pulmonary vasculature, whether directly or indirectly. It is imperative for the radiologist to understand and recognize imaging findings indicating or suggesting pulmonary vascular disease, as the clinical manifestation can be insidious, and for some conditions, early diagnosis and treatment can lead to improved outcomes.

This issue of *Radiologic Clinics of North America* examines the spectrum of pulmonary vascular diseases, ranging from congenital abnormalities to those presenting in childhood and later in life, with attention to the roles imaging plays in both diagnosis and treatment. These talented authors share their expertise with us to further our understanding of this often-challenging topic.

The issue opens with a review of the pathology of pulmonary vascular disease focused on pulmonary hypertension, which is key to understanding the abnormalities encountered in chest imaging. Focused articles explore the spectrum of imaging of pulmonary vascular diseases, including pulmonary hypertension, vasculitis, pulmonary thromboembolism, congenital pulmonary vascular anomalies, neonatal and pediatric pulmonary vascular disease, and pulmonary hypertension, Additional articles discuss the role of cardiovascular MR imaging and interventions in pulmonary vascular disease. The issue concludes with a clinical perspective on the role of imaging in pulmonary vascular disease, a reflection on how essential a multidisciplinary approach is to diagnose these patients.

DISCLOSURE

Consultant, Calyx.ai.

Jeffrey P. Kanne, MD
Department of Radiology
University of Wisconsin School
of Medicine and Public Health
Madison, WI, USA

E-mail address:
JKanne@uwhealth.org

Pathology of Pulmonary Vascular Disease with Radiologic Correlation

Margarita Consing-Gangelhoff, MD[a], Mark Sharobim, MD[a],
Catherine Bodnar, MD[a], Jeffrey P. Kanne, MD[b], Jefree J. Schulte, MD[a],*

KEYWORDS

- Pulmonary hypertension • Pulmonary vasculitis • Pulmonary veno-occlusive disease
- Pulmonary capillary hemangiomatosis • Microscopic polyangiitis • Diffuse alveolar hemorrhage
- ANCA

KEY POINTS

- Pulmonary hypertensive changes result in vascular (usually arterial) remodeling.
- Pulmonary hypertensive changes are mostly nonspecific from a histologic perspective, with a few notable exceptions (plexiform lesions, veno-occlusive disease, and granulomatosis with polyangiitis).
- Pulmonary vascular disease can also be observed in the neonate and posttransplant settings.

INTRODUCTION

Pulmonary vascular disease is typically encountered by the surgical pathologist as a pathologic finding present in the background of some other disease process. A lobectomy for lung cancer or a bullectomy for emphysematous lungs will often show pathologic changes if one goes and examines the vasculature. Most of these changes represent hypertensive changes secondary to some other process, but pathologists may occasionally encounter specimens biopsied or resected for a primary vascular pathology. For simplicity and for the purposes of this review, pulmonary vascular disease is discussed in 4 broad topics: (1) pulmonary hypertension (PAH)—including those conditions arising primary in the lung and changes associated with secondary causes, (2) vasculitis and diffuse alveolar hemorrhage (DAH), (3) congenital and pediatric lesions, and (4) posttransplant vascular changes. The level of detail required to fully discuss the topics in this review deserve standalone articles or individual book chapters, but this is not possible when preparing a succinct review. The discussion of these pathologic entities has been simplified for the purposes of this review and to accommodate the most likely consumer of this review, a radiologist. The main pathologic findings are drawn from numerous other studies and are summarized in this text. The reader is referred to these references and reviews if additional details not covered in this text are desired.[1–5] This article will feature histopathologic changes of PAH and, when applicable, will include corresponding imaging findings, but detailed discussion on imaging will be discussed in subsequent articles.

PULMONARY HYPERTENSION
Introduction

The pulmonary vascular network is characterized by low vascular resistance, typically with pressures one-eighth that of systemic pressures.

---

[a] Department of Pathology and Laboratory Medicine, University of Wisconsin, Madison, WI, USA;
[b] Department of Radiology, University of Wisconsin, Madison, WI, USA
* Corresponding author. Department of Pathology and Laboratory Medicine, University of Wisconsin, 600 Highland Avenue, L5/185, MC 8550, Madison, WI 53792-8550.
E-mail address: jschulte2@wisc.edu

> **Box 1**
> **Pulmonary hypertension division in groups based upon World Health Organization classification**
>
> Group 1: Pulmonary arterial hypertension (PAH)
> Group 2: Pulmonary hypertension due to left heart disease
> Group 3: Pulmonary hypertension due to lung disease and/or hypoxia
> Group 4: Chronic thromboembolic pulmonary hypertension (CTEPH)
> Group 5: Pulmonary hypertension with unclear or multifactorial mechanisms

PAH (PAH will be used throughout this text as the majority of hypertensive change is observed in the pulmonary *arterial* system) is a progressive disease clinically defined as the state in which pressure in the pulmonary artery is increased above a mean of 20 to 25 mm Hg at rest, regardless of the underlying mechanism.[6] It is divided into 5 groups based upon World Health Organization (WHO) classification (Box 1).[7] Patients usually present with symptoms consistent with right ventricular failure such a dyspnea, fatigue, syncope, edema, abdominal pain, and chest pain. In its severe form, PAH may lead to right heart failure and death without adequate treatment. Hypertension in the pulmonary circulation can also occur in physiologic settings, but only transiently, such as with exercise. A recent systematic review based on multinational data by Emmons-Bell and colleagues[8] reported an incidence of 0.0008 to 1.4 cases and prevalence of 0.37 to 15/100,000 person-years.

Radiographic findings of PAH are not uncommonly encountered and are briefly reviewed here.[5,9,10] Classic findings on chest radiographs are usually present in advanced disease: enlarged heart, elevated cardiac apex due to right ventricular hypertrophy, central pulmonary artery dilation, and reduced retrosternal clear space from right ventricular and pulmonary artery enlargement. On chest computed tomography (CT), dilated central and peripheral pulmonary arteries along with end diastolic right ventricular wall thickness less than 4 mm, right ventricular dilation, inferior vena cava and hepatic vein dilation, and centrilobular ground-glass attenuation nodules may be present. Echocardiography is used to assess right ventricular function by measuring systolic pulmonary arterial pressure and tricuspid regurgitation. Cardiac MR imaging is the reference standard for right ventricular function.

The most encountered vascular pathology observed by the practicing surgical pathologist is PAH arising from some secondary process. Most often these are secondary changes observed in the pulmonary arterial system secondary to left heart failure or other conditions. Hypertensive changes are also common in interstitial lung diseases. There are rare cases of primary PAH (now more accurately termed idiopathic PAH), but these are less often seen by the surgical pathologist as primary PAH clinical management has improved in recent years.[11] Pulmonary hypertensive changes may also be observed in the venous system, but conditions that lead to venous hypertension are less commonly observed in surgical pathology. Different histologic classification and grading systems for pulmonary hypertensive change have been developed for PAH (Table 1), but the original grading system is infrequently used in clinical sign-out as many of these histologic changes are rarely encountered, and only grades I, II, and III are seen in standard cases of secondary PAH.[12,13] Regardless of the type of PAH and the

Table 1
Different histologic classification and grading systems for pulmonary hypertensive change for pulmonary hypertension

	Intimal Changes	Medial Changes	Degree of Severity
Grade 1	—	Hypertrophy	Mild-to-moderate pulmonary hypertension
Grade 2	Cellular proliferation	Hypertrophy	
Grade 3	Fibrosis	Hypertrophy; Some vascular dilation	
Grade 4	Fibrosis	Hypertrophy; Progressive dilation	
Grade 5	Fibrosis and plexiform lesions	Hypertrophy; Vascular dilation; and hemosiderin deposition	Severe pulmonary hypertension
Grade 6	Fibrosis and plexiform lesions	Hypertrophy; Vascular dilation; hemosiderin deposition; and necrotizing arteritis	

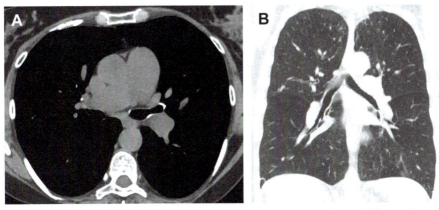

Fig. 1. A 60 year old female individual with chronic obstructive pulmonary disease. (A) Unenhanced CT image shows enlargement of the central pulmonary arteries. (B) Coronal reformatted CT image shows mild hyperinflation with upper lobe predominant emphysema, mild mosaic attenuation, and enlarged central pulmonary arteries.

etiology, destructive remodeling of the vascular bed is observed. These changes are often observed in smaller branches of the pulmonary arteries and consist of either intimal lesions (fibrosis and thickening (**Figs.** 1A, B and 2) or plexiform changes), medial (muscular) hypertrophy/hyperplasia (see **Fig.** 2A, B), or a combination of these changes with or without adventitial changes.[3,4]

Brief Overview of Idiopathic (Primary) Pulmonary Arterial Hypertension

Primary PAH (group 1) includes PAH that arises idiopathically, or from heritable conditions, drugs and/or toxins, or from known associations such as connective tissue diseases, portal hypertension (cirrhosis), or infection (most notably, human immunodeficiency virus). The main histologic finding that separates these forms of PAH from others is the presence of plexiform lesions. While plexiform lesions can be observed across all forms of PAH, their presence strongly suggests a primary (idiopathic) form of PAH. Two other conditions have been classically linked to this group but are distinct from the other conditions in group 1 PAH and show lesions in the venous circulation. These unique conditions include pulmonary veno-occlusive disease (PVOD) and pulmonary capillary hemangiomatosis (PCH). PVOD and PCH both often present with congestive changes and hemosiderin-laden macrophages. Significant fibrous occlusion of veins is diagnostic of PVOD, while capillary proliferations within alveolar septa, near intralobular septa, and near bronchovascular bundles are common in PCH. PVOD and PCH may be seen together, and some view these conditions as a similar disease occurring on a spectrum, which is supported by a more recently described common genetic background of the 2 disease processes.[14–16]

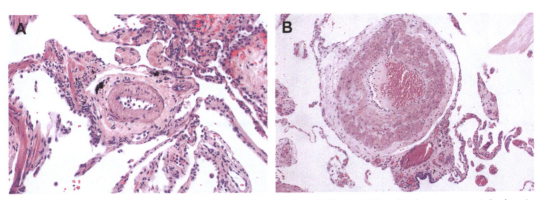

Fig. 2. Histologic findings in areas with emphysema from patient in Fig. 1. (A) Small pulmonary arteriole showing intimal fibrosis (H&E ×200). (B) Small pulmonary artery branch mostly showing medial hypertrophy.

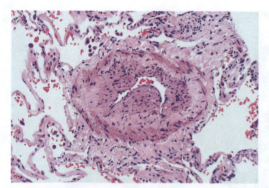

Fig. 3. Severe pulmonary arterial hypertension with narrowing of the lumen by intimal fibrosis (H&E ×200).

Brief Overview of Secondary Pulmonary Arterial Hypertension

Nonidiopathic PAH arises from various secondary processes: left heart disease (group 2), lung diseases and/or hypoxia (group 3), and chronic thromboembolic disease (group 4). Similar to primary PAH (group 1), there is often medial hypertrophy and intimal fibrosis. Muscularization of arterioles and plexiform lesions are typically absent in this group, as are congestive changes and increased numbers of hemosiderin-laden alveolar macrophages.

Pathologic Findings in Pulmonary Hypertension

Nearly all forms of PAH show medial and intimal hyperplasia. In mild-to-moderate PAH, there is medial hypertrophy of medium-sized muscular arteries with some degree of intimal thickening or fibrosis. In severe forms of PAH, there is often significant luminal narrowing from concentric intimal fibrosis (Fig. 3); plexiform and angiomatoid lesions, and necrotizing arteritis, may also be seen in the most severe forms but are not common findings in routine surgical pathology specimens.

While the changes of medial and intimal hyperplasia are present in all forms of PAH, there are subtle clues that can indicate the cause of the PAH. Plexiform (and angiomatoid) lesions (Figs. 4A, B and 5A, B) should prompt the pathologist to consider idiopathic PAH. Plexiform lesions are found in muscular arteries. Plexiform lesions are thought to arise from vascular occlusion, breakdown of elastic layers resulting in endothelial cell proliferation and neolumen formation along with collateralization of vessels.[17,18] Fibrous occlusion of veins (Figs. 6 and 7A, B) is nearly pathognomonic for PVOD. Pulmonary veins are located in the interlobular septa, and occlusion of veins can be quite subtle. Given that there is venous occlusion, this often results in congestion in the arterial system. Congestion is also typical of PCH (Figs. 8A, B and 9A, B). Due to the chronic congestion, it is typical to see numerous intra-alveolar hemosiderin-laden macrophages (Fig. 10) or alveolar hemorrhage. Expert thoracic pathologists often caution rendering a diagnosis of PVOD or PCH in the absence of significant hemosiderin-laden macrophages or hemorrhage. Another secondary cause of PAH that is easily identifiable under the microscope are changes associated with thromboembolic disease. Thromboembolic disease often results in arterial system thrombi (recent fibrin thrombi with or without organization [Figs. 11A, B and 12]), and recanalization (see Fig. 12A, B) can be seen in older lesions. In acute pulmonary embolism (Fig. 13), changes of infarction may also be identified, but this may be a challenging diagnosis in biopsies, due to the multiple pathologic changes that may be observed in infarctions including a pseudogranulomatous response.[19] Eccentric intimal fibrosis is a subtle clue that

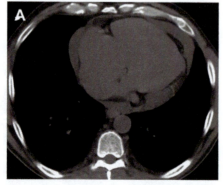
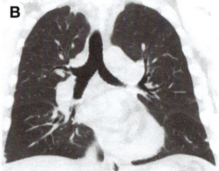

Fig. 4. A 59 year old male patient with idiopathic pulmonary hypertension. (A) Unenhanced CT image shows enlarged right heart chambers and a small pericardial effusion. (B) Coronal reformatted CT image (lung window settings) shows enlarged central pulmonary arteries, which rapidly taper in the periphery.

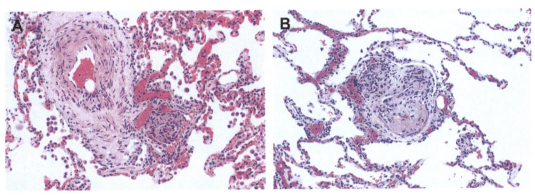

Fig. 5. Histologic findings from same patient as Fig. 4. (A) Small pulmonary artery branch with small neovascular formation along right side of vessel, consistent with plexiform lesion (H&E ×200). (B) Small pulmonary arteriole with plexiform lesion (H&E ×200).

thromboembolic disease may be the cause of PAH. Intravascular foreign material (often easily identified under polarized light), is a form of embolic disease, often seen in patients with a history of intravenous (IV) drug use. A similar phenomena to IV drug use is the recent identification of hydrophilic polymer in the vascular system following numerous intravascular cannulations (Fig. 14).[20,21]

VASCULITIS AND DIFFUSE ALVEOLAR HEMORRHAGE
Introduction

Vasculitis and DAH are distinct clinicopathologic entities but will be discussed together here as they may be encountered together. In its simplest definition, DAH is a form of acute lung injury manifesting with hemorrhage that fills the alveolar air spaces.[22] DAH is not always a result of a vasculitic process and can be encountered in a surgical

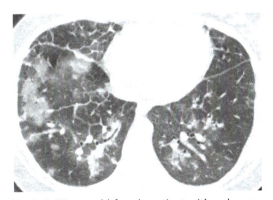

Fig. 6. A 35 year old female patient with pulmonary veno-occlusive disease/pulmonary capillary hemangiomatosis. Unenhanced CT image shows diffuse septal thickening with patchy ground-glass opacity reflecting distended pulmonary veins and edema.

pathology specimen from a patient with infection, malignancy, or any form of acute lung injury. Nonetheless, in patients with DAH, one should examine the specimen carefully for evidence of capillaritis and/or vasculitis given that these conditions may also give rise to DAH. DAH is often observed in granulomatosis with polyangiitis (GPA) and microscopic polyangiitis (MPA), in the setting of pulmonary involvement by underlying collagen vascular diseases, and among other conditions.

Entities Presenting with Diffuse Alveolar Hemorrhage/Vasculitis and Their Associated Pathologic Findings

When assessing for hemorrhagic processes in the lung, it is important to remember that the lung is a highly vascular organ with both pulmonary arterial and systemic blood supply. Each airway is paired with a corresponding branch of the pulmonary artery. Thus, it is common to encounter blood, or recent hemorrhage, in a lung specimen when viewed under the microscope. A common pitfall, especially of less experienced pathologists, is the overcalling of procedural hemorrhage as DAH. There are clues one can use to separate recent procedural or artifactual hemorrhage from pathologic DAH. Procedural hemorrhage often contains numerous neutrophils and other formed elements of blood and does not typically contain significant amounts of fibrin or hemosiderin laden macrophages. On the contrary, if one is to encounter red blood cells admixed with fibrin and/or the presence of alveolar septal capillaritis, a diagnosis of DAH (Figs. 15 and 16A, B) may be considered.

GPA is a small (including capillaries) to medium-sized vessel, antineutrophil cytoplasmic antibodies (ANCA)-associated vasculitis.[23] It presents as

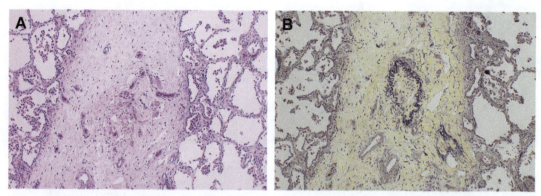

Fig. 7. Histologic findings from the patient in **Fig. 6**. (*A*) Interlobular septum with subtle finding of occluded pulmonary vein (H&E ×100). (*B*) Special stains for elastic fibers (*black*) outline the vein elastic lamina, highlighting the lumen is occluded (Movat pentachrome stain ×100).

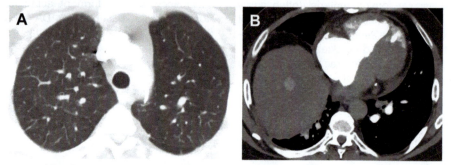

Fig. 8. A 56 year old male patient with pulmonary capillary hemangiomatosis. (*A*) Contrast-enhanced CT image (lung window settings) shows enlarged peripheral pulmonary arteries, mild mosaic attenuation, and minimal septal thickening. (*B*) Contrast-enhanced CT image shows right ventricular hypertrophy, right atrial enlargement, and dilated peripheral pulmonary arteries.

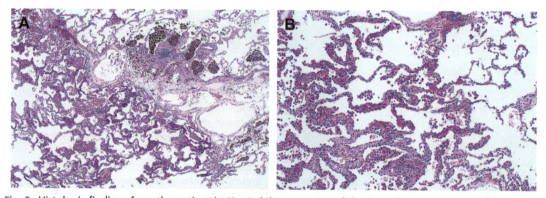

Fig. 9. Histologic findings from the patient in **Fig. 8**. (*A*) Low power of the lung shows thickened alveolar septa and vascular congestion, most prominent in the lower left field. This capillary proliferation is adjacent to an interlobular septum, a common location to see changes of pulmonary capillary hemangiomatosis (H&E ×40). (*B*) Higher power images show capillary proliferation and congestion in affected alveolar septa (*left side*) contrasted by normal alveoli (*right side*; H&E ×100).

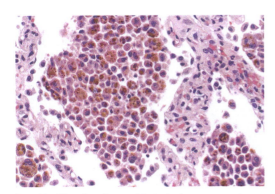

Fig. 10. Alveolar hemosiderin-laden macrophages. This finding is common in pulmonary veno-occlusive disease and pulmonary capillary hemangiomatosis, as well as diffuse alveolar hemorrhage (H&E ×400).

necrotizing granulomatous inflammation affecting the upper and lower respiratory tracts and as a necrotizing vasculitis. Necrotizing glomerulonephritis, ocular vasculitis, and pulmonary vasculitis with hemorrhage are additional common presentations. It is predominantly associated with cANCA/PR-3 ANCA antibodies, with fewer than 5% of cases having myeloperoxidase (MPO) ANCA antibodies.[24,25] The incidence of GPA is estimated to be approximately 9.8 cases per million people per year with a prevalence of 23.7 cases per million people.[26,27] The median age of diagnosis is 68 years, predominantly in Northern European individuals.[26–28] Histologic features include a necrotizing, granulomatous inflammation consisting of palisading histiocytes and occasional giant cells, with fibrinoid necrosis of vessels (Fig. 17).[29] The necrosis is often described as "dirty" with abundant cellular debris. Approximately 60% of patients with pulmonary capillaritis have GPA, which can lead to DAH.[23,30]

MPA is a small and medium vessel, ANCA-associated vasculitis.[23] The pathophysiology involves neutrophil exposure to proinflammatory cytokines, which then leads to neutrophil surface expression of MPO.[31] This attracts antibodies (MPO-ANCA) that then activate neutrophils and complement causing vessel wall inflammation and damage.[31] Necrotizing glomerulonephritis is a common presentation.[23] The incidence of MPA is estimated to be about 10.1 cases per million people per year with a prevalence of 25.1 cases per million people.[26,27] The median age of diagnosis is 70 years.[26] Histologic features include a necrotizing vasculitis, without granulomatous inflammation, mostly affecting small vessels.[23] About 3% of patients with pulmonary capillaritis can have MPA, which can lead to DAH.[23,26,27,30,31] There is acute hemorrhage with hemosiderin-laden macrophages in alveolar spaces, and necrotizing capillaritis can also be observed.[30]

The collagen vascular diseases that most often affect the pulmonary system include rheumatoid arthritis (RA), progressive systemic sclerosis, systemic lupus erythematosus (SLE), polymyositis and dermatomyositis, mixed connective tissue disease, and Sjögren syndrome.[32,33] pANCA can be associated in up to 30% of patients with SLE or RA and in less than 5% of other connective tissue diseases, without specificity for PR3 or MPO.[24] Alveolar hemorrhage, a rare complication in SLE, and PAH are manifestations.[34] A total of 11% of patients with pulmonary capillaritis have systemic autoimmune disease including RA and SLE.[34] About 2% of patients with SLE have pulmonary vasculitis attributed to their chronic disease.[35] Pulmonary capillaritis and vasculitis are rare in both mixed connective tissue disease and systemic sclerosis, respectively.[36,37] Histologic findings include fresh hemorrhage, intra-alveolar

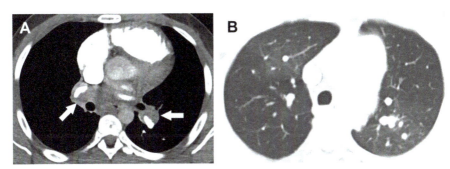

Fig. 11. A 24 year old male patient with chronic thromboembolic pulmonary hypertension. (A) Contrast-enhanced CT image shows dilated lower lobe pulmonary arteries with eccentric filling defects (arrows). (B) Contrast-enhanced CT image (lung window settings) shows mosaic attenuation characterized by areas of increased attenuation with large vessels, areas of normal attenuation with normal vessels, and areas of low attenuation with small vessels.

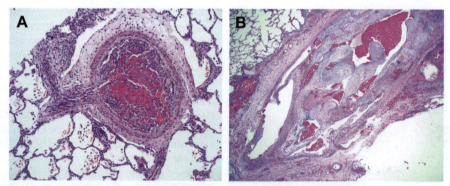

Fig. 12. Histologic findings from the patient in Fig. 11. (*A*) Medium-sized pulmonary artery with recent thrombus. The lumen of the artery is filled with blood, fibrin, and other formed elements of blood (H&E ×100). (*B*) Large central lung artery with remote infarction that has been recanalized (H&E ×20).

fibrin, and hemosiderin-laden macrophages.[36] There is necrotizing capillaritis consisting of neutrophils with necrotic debris within intra-alveolar septa.[36] Arteritis in SLE reveals transmural inflammation and fibrinoid necrosis.[35] Foci of fibrinoid necrosis are seen in systemic sclerosis as well.[37]

Eosinophilic granulomatosis with polyangiitis (EGPA) is a small and medium vessel, ANCA-associated vasculitis.[23] It commonly affects the respiratory tract and is associated with asthma and eosinophilia.[23] Nasal polyps are a typical presentation.[23] There can be nongranulomatous eosinophil-rich inflammation of the lungs, heart, and gastrointestinal tract.[23]

The incidence of EGPA is estimated to be about 0.9 cases per million people per year with a prevalence of 10.7 cases per million people.[26,27] The median age of diagnosis is 61 years.[27]

Histologic features include an eosinophil-predominant necrotizing granulomatous inflammation, eosinophilic pneumonia, and leukocytoclastic vasculitis.[23,38,39] There may be alveolar hemorrhage with fresh blood, hemosiderin-laden macrophages in the interstitium, and a necrotizing vasculitis.[30]

Radiographic Correlates Observed in Diffuse Alveolar Hemorrhage/Vasculitis

CT is the preferred examination for evaluating the lungs for vasculitis and DAH. In GPA, nodules, masses, and cavities are common with more extensive consolidation and ground-glass opacity (GGO) in DAH.[40] Consolidation and GGO are common with MPA and anti-glomerular basememt membrane (GBM) disease.[41] In antiphopholipid syndrome (APS), chest radiograph and CT can show bilateral multifocal lung consolidation, particularly when associated with acute respiratory distress syndrome.[42] In EGPA, chest radiographic findings include patchy, sometimes migratory consolidation. On CT, peripheral and peribronchial GGO and consolidation may be present. Additionally, centrilobular nodules, bronchial wall

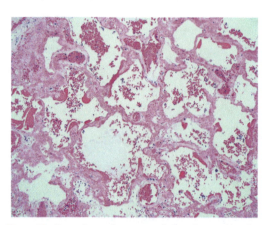

Fig. 13. Recent pulmonary infarction showing ghosted alveoli lacking basophilia due to lack of nuclear staining secondary to cell death (H&E ×100).

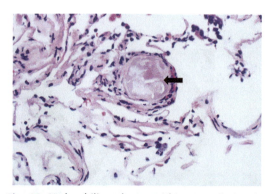

Fig. 14. Hydrophilic polymer within a small alveolar capillary (*arrow*). This is a lung transplant patient with multiple intravascular procedures. In this case, there was no associated signs of infarction, and this was an incidental findings on lung transplant surveillance biopsy (H&E ×400).

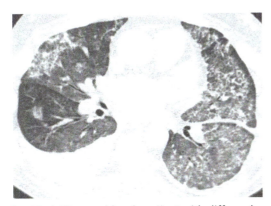

Fig. 15. A 72 year old male patient with diffuse alveolar hemorrhage. Unenhanced CT image shows extensive ground-glass opacity admixed with small foci of consolidation. There is relative subpleural sparing on the left and a small layering right pleural effusion.

thickening, and interlobular septal thickening may be present. Pleural effusions can develop in the setting of eosinophilic pleuritis or eosinophilic cardiomyopathy-related congestive heart failure.[39]

CONGENITAL AND PEDIATRIC LESIONS

While there are other entities that affect the neonatal and childhood lung, alveolar capillary dysplasia with misalignment of pulmonary veins (ACD/MPV) deserves discussion here. ACD/MPV is a newborn interstitial lung disease, characterized by abnormal alveolar capillary formation that disrupts the normal blood-gas exchange.[43,44] Anomalous pulmonary veins are also present.[43,44] Patients are divided into typical and atypical groups, with the typical group presenting with hypoxemic respiratory failure and death within a few hours after birth, while atypical cases survive beyond the neonatal period.[43] ACD/MPV is associated with mutations in *FoxF1* in up to 60% of cases.[45] ACD/MPV is a rare, lethal disease, with more than 200 cases reported since it was first described in 1981.[43,44]

Bronchi, bronchioles, and arteries have normal branching, but alveolar walls are atypically widened by loose mesenchyme with a prominent myxoid matrix.[44] Capillaries are decreased in number and are centrally located (**Figs. 18**A, B and **19**), lacking communication with the alveolar epithelium, which can be highlighted by CD31.[43,44] Muscularized arterioles are seen in alveolar walls, which should not be present past bronchioles in normal neonatal lung, due to PAH.[44] Abnormal vein location and drainage is noted.[44] Veins appear to run with muscular pulmonary arteries, within bronchial arteriolar sheaths (see **Fig. 19**A, B).[43,44] Additionally, there can be small vessel congestion.[43] Atypical cases appear to have mixed features of normal lung and classic histology of ACD/MPV.[44] Radiographic correlates of ACD/MPV in the chest radiograph can show patchy lung opacities but normal lung volumes.[44]

POSTTRANSPLANT VASCULAR COMPLICATIONS

There are 2 major vascular complications that are observed in the lung allograft. In the postoperative period, numerous complications can arise with the arterial and venous anastomoses.[46] There can be kinking of the vessels, thrombus, or luminal narrowing (stricture). Anastomotic complications are associated with high morbidity and mortality. The other major complication of the posttransplant pulmonary vasculature is chronic vascular rejection (vasculopathy).[47] There is intimal fibrosis and vascular thickening (**Fig. 20**). Allograft vasculopathy is usually observed in large resections or explants of lung allografts along with bronchiolitis obliterans.

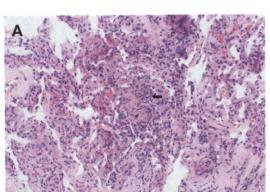
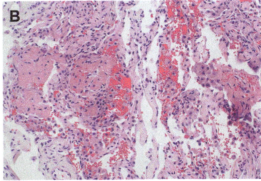

Fig. 16. Histologic findings from the patient in Fig. 15. (A) Organizing blood and fibrin (*asterisk*) with increased alveolar septal cellularity (*arrow*) suggestive of capillaritis (H&E ×200). (B) Another section of alveolated lung parenchyma showing red blood cells admixed with fibrin, without a significant interstitial infiltrate (H&E ×200).

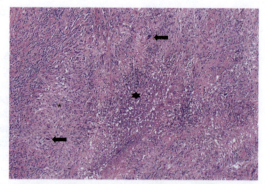

Fig. 17. Histologic findings of granulomatosis with polyangiitis. There is destruction of a pulmonary artery branch with dirty necrosis (*star*), a rim of epithelioid histiocytes (*asterisk*), and scattered multinucleated giant cells (*arrows*; H&E ×100).

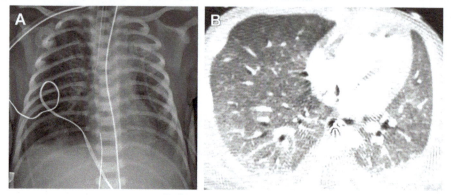

Fig. 18. A 3 day old female infant with alveolar capillary dysplasia. (*A*) AP radiograph shows a diffuse granular appearance of the lungs. (*B*) Unenhanced CT image shows diffuse ground-glass opacity.

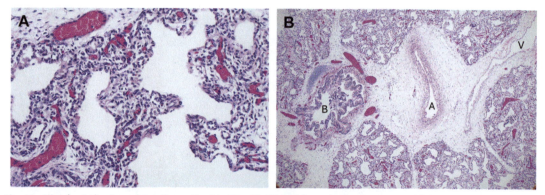

Fig. 19. Histologic findings from the patient in **Fig. 18**. (*A*) Thickened alveolar septa with loose mesenchymal matrix supporting centrally located alveolar capillaries (H&E ×200). (*B*) Bronchovascular sheath containing the airway (B), pulmonary artery (A), and an anomalously located vein (V; H&E ×20).

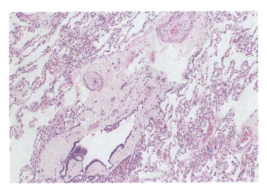

Fig. 20. Allograft vasculopathy characterized by luminal narrow of pulmonary arterioles, mostly by intimal fibrosis. Note that the corresponding airway shows subepithelial fibrosis compatible with bronchiolitis obliterans (H&E, ×100).

SUMMARY

In summary, pulmonary vascular changes are commonly observed by the pulmonary pathologist, and the majority of these changes are nonspecific and due to secondary processes. Primary (idiopathic) pulmonary vascular changes often include more severe or extreme changes including plexiform lesions and pulmonary venous occlusion. Vasculitis and capillaritis can be seen in surgical pathology specimens and are often associated with ANCA-vasculitis or collagen vascular disease. Specific vascular changes can also be observed in the neonate and posttransplant setting.

CLINICS CARE POINTS

- Pulmonary hypertensive changes in the lung always result in destructive remodeling of the vascular bed.
- Pulmonary hypertensive changes most often result in a combination of intimal and medial changes.
- Plexiform lesions are more commonly associated with idiopathic and severe forms of PAH.
- PVOD and PCH often occur as a spectrum of changes and show unique pathologic changes.
- Vasculitis, capillaritis, and DAH often overlap and can be seen as a part of systemic ANCA-associated vasculitis or collagen vascular disease.
- ACD/MPV shows unique diagnostic changes including centrally located alveolar capillaries and pulmonary veins in proximity to pulmonary arteries.
- Chronic lung allograft vasculopathy is a vascular change observed in lung allograft with chronic lung allograft dysfunction/chronic rejection.

DISCLOSURE

The authors have nothing to disclose.

REFERENCES

1. Katzenstein A-LA. Diagnostic atlas of non-neoplastic lung disease: a practical guide for surgical pathologists. 1st edition. New York: Springer Publishing Company; 2016.
2. Mukhopadhyay S. Non-neoplastic pulmonary pathology: an algorithmic approach to histologic findings in the lung. United Kingdom: Cambridge University Press; 2016.
3. Tuder RM, Marecki JC, Richter A, et al. Pathology of pulmonary hypertension. Clin Chest Med 2007; 28(1):23–42, vii.
4. Humbert M, Guignabert C, Bonnet S, et al. Pathology and pathobiology of pulmonary hypertension: state of the art and research perspectives. Eur Respir J 2019;53(1):1801887.
5. Peña E, Dennie C, Veinot J, et al. Pulmonary hypertension: how the radiologist can help. Radiographics 2012;32(1):9–32.
6. Maron BA. Revised definition of pulmonary hypertension and approach to management: a clinical primer. J Am Heart Assoc 2023;12(8):e029024.
7. Simonneau G, Gatzoulis MA, Adatia I, et al. Updated clinical classification of pulmonary hypertension. J Am Coll Cardiol 2013;62(25 Suppl):D34–41.
8. Emmons-Bell S, Johnson C, Boon-Dooley A, et al. Prevalence, incidence, and survival of pulmonary arterial hypertension: a systematic review for the global burden of disease 2020 study. Pulm Circ 2022;12(1):e12020.
9. Goerne H, Batra K, Rajiah P. Imaging of pulmonary hypertension: an update. Cardiovasc Diagn Ther 2018;8(3):279–96.
10. Altschul E, Remy-Jardin M, Machnicki S, et al. Imaging of pulmonary hypertension: pictorial essay. Chest 2019;156(2):211–27.
11. Sahay S, Chakinala MM, Kim NH, et al. Contemporary treatment of pulmonary arterial hypertension: a US perspective. Am J Respir Crit Care Med 2024; 210(5):581–92.
12. Heath D, Edwards JE. The pathology of hypertensive pulmonary vascular disease; a description of six grades of structural changes in the pulmonary arteries with special reference to congenital cardiac septal defects. Circulation 1958;18(4 Part 1): 533–47.

13. Wagenvoort CA. Grading of pulmonary vascular lesions–a reappraisal. Histopathology 1981;5(6):595–8.
14. Park JE, Chang SA, Jang SY, et al. Differential diagnosis of pulmonary veno-occlusive disease and/or pulmonary capillary hemangiomatosis after identification of two novel EIF2AK4 variants by whole-exome sequencing. Mol Syndromol 2023;14(3):254–7.
15. Emanuelli G, Zhu J, Li W, et al. Functional validation of EIF2AK4 (GCN2) missense variants associated with pulmonary arterial hypertension. Hum Mol Genet 2024;33(17):1495–505.
16. Weatherald J, Dorfmüller P, Perros F, et al. Pulmonary capillary haemangiomatosis: a distinct entity? Eur Respir Rev 2020;29(156):190168.
17. Cool CD, Stewart JS, Werahera P, et al. Three-dimensional reconstruction of pulmonary arteries in plexiform pulmonary hypertension using cell-specific markers. Evidence for a dynamic and heterogeneous process of pulmonary endothelial cell growth. Am J Pathol 1999;155(2):411–9.
18. Rajagopal S, Yu YA. The pathobiology of pulmonary arterial hypertension. Cardiol Clin 2022;40(1):1–12.
19. Yousem SA. The surgical pathology of pulmonary infarcts: diagnostic confusion with granulomatous disease, vasculitis, and neoplasia. Mod Pathol 2009;22(5):679–85.
20. Mehta RI, Mehta RI, Chun Y. Hydrophilic polymer embolism: an underrecognized iatrogenic cause of ischemia, inflammation, and coagulopathy. Hum Pathol 2015;46(3):488–9.
21. Chopra AM, Mehta M, Bismuth J, et al. Polymer coating embolism from intravascular medical devices - a clinical literature review. Cardiovasc Pathol 2017;30:45–54.
22. Hughes KT, Beasley MB. Pulmonary manifestations of acute lung injury: more than just diffuse alveolar damage. Arch Pathol Lab Med 2017;141(7):916–22.
23. Jennette JC, Falk RJ, Bacon PA, et al. 2012 revised international chapel hill consensus conference nomenclature of vasculitides. Arthritis Rheum 2013;65(1):1–11.
24. Schönermarck U, Lamprecht P, Csernok E, et al. Prevalence and spectrum of rheumatic diseases associated with proteinase 3-antineutrophil cytoplasmic antibodies (ANCA) and myeloperoxidase-ANCA. Rheumatology (Oxford) 2001;40(2):178–84.
25. Hoffman GS, Kerr GS, Leavitt RY, et al. Wegener granulomatosis: an analysis of 158 patients. Ann Intern Med 1992;116(6):488–98.
26. Mohammad AJ, Jacobsson LT, Westman KW, et al. Incidence and survival rates in Wegener's granulomatosis, microscopic polyangiitis, Churg-Strauss syndrome and polyarteritis nodosa. Rheumatology (Oxford) 2009;48(12):1560–5.
27. Mahr A, Guillevin L, Poissonnet M, et al. Prevalences of polyarteritis nodosa, microscopic polyangiitis, Wegener's granulomatosis, and Churg-Strauss syndrome in a French urban multiethnic population in 2000: a capture-recapture estimate. Arthritis Rheum 2004;51(1):92–9.
28. Terrier B, Dechartres A, Deligny C, et al. Granulomatosis with polyangiitis according to geographic origin and ethnicity: clinical-biological presentation and outcome in a French population. Rheumatology (Oxford) 2017;56(3):445–50.
29. Devaney KO, Travis WD, Hoffman G, et al. Interpretation of head and neck biopsies in Wegener's granulomatosis. A pathologic study of 126 biopsies in 70 patients. Am J Surg Pathol 1990;14(6):555–64.
30. Thompson G, Klecka M, Roden AC, et al. Biopsy-proven pulmonary capillaritis: a retrospective study of aetiologies including an in-depth look at isolated pulmonary capillaritis. Respirology 2016;21(4):734–8.
31. Xiao H, Schreiber A, Heeringa P, et al. Alternative complement pathway in the pathogenesis of disease mediated by anti-neutrophil cytoplasmic autoantibodies. Am J Pathol 2007;170(1):52–64.
32. Capobianco J, Grimberg A, Thompson BM, et al. Thoracic manifestations of collagen vascular diseases. Radiographics 2012;32(1):33–50.
33. Schulte JJ, Husain AN. Connective tissue disease related interstitial lung disease. Surg Pathol Clin 2020;13(1):165–88.
34. Jawad H, McWilliams SR, Bhalla S. Cardiopulmonary manifestations of collagen vascular diseases. Curr Rheumatol Rep 2017;19(11):71.
35. Haupt HM, Moore GW, Hutchins GM. The lung in systemic lupus erythematosus. Analysis of the pathologic changes in 120 patients. Am J Med 1981;71(5):791–8.
36. Schwarz MI, Zamora MR, Hodges TN, et al. Isolated pulmonary capillaritis and diffuse alveolar hemorrhage in rheumatoid arthritis and mixed connective tissue disease. Chest 1998;113(6):1609–15.
37. Griffin MT, Robb JD, Martin JR. Diffuse alveolar haemorrhage associated with progressive systemic sclerosis. Thorax 1990;45(11):903–4.
38. Kawakami T, Soma Y, Kawasaki K, et al. Initial cutaneous manifestations consistent with mononeuropathy multiplex in Churg-Strauss syndrome. Arch Dermatol 2005;141(7):873–8.
39. Kim YK, Lee KS, Chung MP, et al. Pulmonary involvement in Churg-Strauss syndrome: an analysis of CT, clinical, and pathologic findings. Eur Radiol 2007;17(12):3157–65.
40. Papiris SA, Manoussakis MN, Drosos AA, et al. Imaging of thoracic Wegener's granulomatosis: the computed tomographic appearance. Am J Med 1992;93(5):529–36.
41. Guggenberger KV, Bley TA. Imaging in vasculitis. Curr Rheumatol Rep 2020;22(8):34.
42. Espinosa G, Cervera R, Font J, et al. The lung in the antiphospholipid syndrome. Ann Rheum Dis 2002;61(3):195–8.

43. Alturkustani M, Li D, Byers JT, et al. Histopathologic features of alveolar capillary dysplasia with misalignment of pulmonary veins with atypical clinical presentation. Cardiovasc Pathol 2021;50:107289.
44. Janney CG, Askin FB, Kuhn C 3rd. Congenital alveolar capillary dysplasia–an unusual cause of respiratory distress in the newborn. Am J Clin Pathol 1981; 76(5):722–7.
45. Szafranski P, Gambin T, Dharmadhikari AV, et al. Pathogenetics of alveolar capillary dysplasia with misalignment of pulmonary veins. Hum Genet 2016;135(5):569–86.
46. Siddique A, Bose AK, Özalp F, et al. Vascular anastomotic complications in lung transplantation: a single institution's experience. Interact Cardiovasc Thorac Surg 2013;17(4):625–31.
47. Stewart S, Fishbein MC, Snell GI, et al. Revision of the 1996 working formulation for the standardization of nomenclature in the diagnosis of lung rejection. J Heart Lung Transplant 2007;26(12):1229–42.

Imaging Approach to Pulmonary Hypertension

Shravan Sridhar, MD, MS[a],*, Sayedomid Ebrahimzadeh, MD[b,c], Hannah Ahn, MD[c,d], Christopher Lee, MD[c], Jonathan Liu, MD, MS[a]

KEYWORDS

- Pulmonary hypertension • WHO groups • Chest CT • Radiography

KEY POINTS

- Pulmonary hypertension can cause significant morbidity and mortality.
- Diagnosis of pulmonary hypertension proceeds stepwise, with tests ordered to exclude the most to least common causes of pulmonary hypertension.
- Pulmonary hypertension is classified into 5 groups in the World Health Organization (WHO) classification.
- Patients can have pulmonary hypertension from more than one WHO group.
- Chest computed tomography is useful in evaluating for conditions in all 5 WHO groups.

INTRODUCTION

Pulmonary hypertension (PH) is a pathologic state characterized by elevated pressure in the pulmonary arteries and sometimes the pulmonary veins. If left untreated, PH can lead to significant morbidity and mortality. Epidemiologic data on PH of all causes are sparse. One population-based cohort study in Canada showed the annual incidence and prevalence to be 0.029% and 0.127% in 2012, respectively.[1] Interestingly, this represented an increase in incidence and prevalence by 20% and 28%, respectively, from 2002.[1]

Suspicion for PH may arise from abnormal clinical presentation or incidental detection of secondary features of PH on diagnostic testing. When there is sufficient concern, a diagnostic workup is pursued to first confirm a diagnosis of PH and followed by determination of the underlying cause. Imaging plays an important role in the detection, diagnosis, and management of PH. It is important for radiologists to recognize the underlying causes of PH and their respective imaging findings because identification of these patients allows for initiation of treatment strategies to mitigate the detrimental effects of longstanding PH. The following discussion will focus on the evaluation of PH, utility of imaging, and imaging appearance of common causes of PH.

DEFINITION OF PULMONARY HYPERTENSION

PH occurs with elevated pulmonary vascular resistance and pulmonary artery pressure, which may be caused by 1 or more factors including abnormalities of pulmonary blood flow and cardiac function, hypoxic vasoconstriction, or exposure to toxins or metabolites.

Sustained elevation of the mean pulmonary artery pressure (mPAP) is diagnostic of PH. Normal mPAP is 14 ± 3 mm Hg at rest and mPAP greater than 20 mm Hg is considered elevated.[2] Previously, PH was defined by an mPAP ≥25 mm Hg, with mPAP of 21 to 24 mm Hg classified as borderline PH, necessitating further evaluation.[3,4] However, increasing evidence has shown greater mortality in

---

[a] Department of Radiology and Biomedical Imaging, University of California San Francisco, M-391 Box 0628, 505 Parnassus Avenue, San Francisco, CA 94143, USA; [b] Department of Radiology, University of British Columbia, 899 W 12th Avenue, Vancouver, BC V5Z1M9, Canada; [c] Department of Cardiology, University of California San Francisco, M-310 Box 0214, 505 Parnassus Avenue, San Francisco, CA 94143, USA; [d] Department of Radiology, San Antonio Military Medical Center, 1100 Wilford Hall Loop, JBSA-Lackland, TX 78236, USA
* Corresponding author.
E-mail address: Shravan.Sridhar@ucsf.edu

patients with mPAP of 21 to 24 mm Hg compared to those with mPAP ≤20 mm Hg.[5] As a result, the 2022 European Society of Cardiology /European Respiratory Society Guidelines for the diagnosis and treatment of PH reclassified mPAP greater than 20 mm Hg as diagnostic of PH.[6,7]

CLASSIFICATION OF PULMONARY HYPERTENSION

The World Health Organization (WHO) classification of PH is the most widely recognized and used classification system for the diagnosis and management of patients with PH (**Table 1**). This system divides cases of PH into 5 groups based on underlying etiology and is helpful for offering insight into potential management strategies.

DIAGNOSTIC EVALUATION OF PULMONARY HYPERTENSION

PH is sometimes discovered during an investigation into the cause of various symptoms such as progressive shortness of breath, chest pressure/pain, and dizziness.[8,9] Due to the nonspecific nature of these symptoms and insidious onset, there is often a diagnostic delay of about 2 years from initial onset of symptoms, often longer in younger patients.[10] Once clinical suspicion for PH is raised, several diagnostic tests are performed including pulmonary function testing, arterial blood gases, and various blood tests such as complete blood count and human immunodeficiency virus assay. Additional laboratory tests may be considered in select cases, such as connective tissue disease serologies. Finally, a variety of imaging tests are used.

As left heart failure is the most common cause of PH,[1] echocardiography is often the first diagnostic examination in the evaluation of PH. Beyond cardiac function, echocardiography can detect secondary features suggestive of PH such as right ventricular hypertrophy or dilation as well as indirectly estimate pulmonary arterial pressures.[11,12] In select cases, cardiac MR imaging can be used to assess cardiac function and morphology and

Table 1				
World Health Organization classification of pulmonary hypertension				
World Health Organization (WHO) Group	Disorders	Pathogenesis	Radiologic Imaging	Treatment Approach
1	Idiopathic, heritable, substance-induced, CTD, human immunodeficiency virus, portal hypertension, simple cardiovascular shunts, PVOD, PCH	Proliferative vasculopathy affecting pre-capillary pulmonary arterioles or venules	Chest computed tomography	Vasodilators, treatment of underlying problem (eg, congenital heart disease)
2	Left heart failure, valvular heart disease	Pulmonary venous hypertension due to poor forward flow	Cardiac CT/MR imaging in specific cases	Treatment of heart failure or heart transplant
3	Lung disease, hypoxia	Poorly understood pathogenesis	High-resolution chest CT	Treatment of lung disease or lung transplant
4	Pulmonary artery obstruction	Mechanical flow obstruction	Chest computed tomography angiography (CTA)	Removal of pulmonary artery obstruction
5	Hematologic disorders, metabolic disorders, complex CHD	Multifactorial or idiopathic	Chest CT/CTA Cardiac CT/MR imaging	Treatment of underlying factors, vasodilators may be considered

Of the 5 groups, WHO Group 1 has the most varied underlying etiologies. Disitinguishing among the different WHO groups requires a comprehensive evaluation including but not limited to echocardiography, right heart catheterization, and chest CT. Patients can have pulmonary hypertension due to disorders from more than 1 WHO group.

Abbreviations: CTD, connective tissue disease; CHD, congenital heart disease; PVOD, pulmonary veno-occlusive disease; PCH, pulmonary capillary hemangiomatosis.

to detect underlying cardiomyopathies contributing to or causing PH.[13]

The second most common cause of PH is chronic lung disease.[1] As a result, chest radiographs and noncontrast chest computed tomography (CT) are often performed early in the evaluation of PH to identify chronic lung conditions such as chronic obstructive pulmonary disease (COPD) and fibrotic interstitial lung disease (ILD), which are associated with development of PH.[14–16] Noncontrast chest CT enables accurate characterization of the severity and extent of lung disease if present.

If cardiac and pulmonary parenchymal causes are not thought to be the cause of PH, ventilation-perfusion scan and CT pulmonary angiography are performed to evaluate for pulmonary artery obstructions.

If noninvasive testing does not reveal a cause for PH, right heart catheterization (RHC) can confirm a diagnosis of WHO Group 1 PH. Furthermore, RHC offers the ability to measure the (mPAP) and determine whether the patient has pre-capillary and/or post-capillary PH as well as ascertain disease severity. Becoming familiar with the results of RHC is helpful for understanding potential causes of PH (**Table 2**).

APPROACH TO PULMONARY HYPERTENSION ON RADIOLOGIC IMAGING

Although knowing the typical sequence of diagnostic testing for PH is helpful, the etiology is not always clear. Patients do not always fall under a single WHO Group. Furthermore, suspicion for PH may be raised either through clinical assessment or through imaging. As such, the role the radiologist plays can differ depending on the stage of the diagnostic evaluation.

Because chest radiographs and CT are the most common initial imaging tests performed in patients being evaluated for PH, the remainder of this article will focus on these 2 modalities and potential findings signaling specific causes of PH.

CHEST RADIOGRAPHY

Chest radiography is a first-line imaging test to evaluate for signs of PH and detect overt heart or lung disease as a potential etiology. Features of PH on chest radiography include dilation of the main, hilar, and intrapulmonary pulmonary arteries, vascular pruning, pronounced definition of intrapulmonary vascular margins, and right atrial and ventricular dilation (**Fig. 1**). Heart disease can manifest with cardiac silhouette enlargement and pulmonary edema, which can be suggested by indistinct vascular margins, increased central pulmonary vascular caliber, vascular redistribution, Kerley B lines, perihilar opacities, and pleural effusion. Pulmonary causes of PH are grouped into obstructive and restrictive lung diseases. Obstructive lung disease such as COPD can produce pulmonary hyperlucency and hyperinflation, with widening of the AP thoracic diameter and flattening of the diaphragm. Restrictive lung disease such as pulmonary fibrosis can cause coarse reticular opacities, traction bronchiectasis, architectural distortion, and reduced lung volume. Further characterization of these findings is performed with chest CT.

CHEST COMPUTED TOMOGRAPHY

The typical protocol for a comprehensive evaluation of ILD is a helical scan from the clavicles through the diaphragm with less than 1.5 mm axial reconstructions in sharp and soft tissue kernels

Table 2
Hemodynamic classification of pulmonary hypertension

Hemodynamic Type	Right Heart Catheterization Metrics	WHO Group
Precapillary	Pulmonary venous hypertension: Absent Pulmonary vascular resistance: High	1, 3, 4, 5
Postcapillary	Pulmonary venous hypertension: Present Pulmonary vascular resistance: Low	2, 5
Precapillary and postcapillary	Pulmonary venous hypertension: Present Pulmonary vascular resistance: High	2, 5

Right heart catheterization metrics can be used to include or exclude different types of pulmonary hypertension. A high pulmonary capillary wedge pressure (PCWP) suggests post-capillary pulmonary hypertension. Pulmonary vascular resistance (PVR) is calculated using the PCWP, mean pulmonary artery pressure (mPAP), and cardiac output. High PVR suggests pre-capillary pulmonary hypertension. While right heart catheterization is most helpful in including or excluding a component of WHO Group 2 pulmonary hypertension, it is less helpful in discerning between the remaining types of pulmonary hypertension, where cross-sectional imaging plays a critical role.

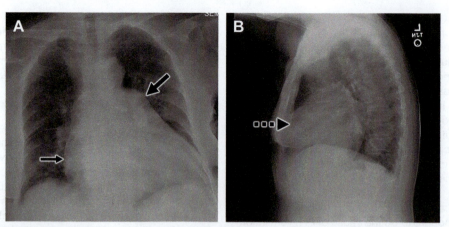

Fig. 1. Features of pulmonary hypertension on chest radiography. (*A*) A frontal chest radiograph of a 76-year-old woman with pulmonary hypertension shows dilated main pulmonary artery (*thick arrow*) and right atrium (*thin arrow*). (*B*) Lateral chest radiograph shows dilated right ventricle (*dashed arrow*) occupying a larger space, particularly in the craniocaudal dimension, resulting in effacement and craniocaudal shortening of the retrosternal clear space.

with coronal and sagittal multiplanar reformats. Additionally, expiratory imaging, either static or dynamic, is necessary to assess for air trapping. Depending on institutional protocol or ordering physician preference, intravenous contrast may or may not be administered for the examination. If evaluation of the pulmonary arteries in the setting of chronic thromboembolic disease is desired, it is advisable to perform the study using bolus tracking with the trigger region of interest (ROI) placed on the main pulmonary artery, with trigger threshold set to 150 to 200 Hounsfield unit (HU), or on the left atrium with a trigger threshold set to blood pool + 60 HU to ensure adequate enhancement of the pulmonary arteries. The next sections discuss the typical findings of PH grouped by organ system.

VASCULAR FINDINGS
Pulmonary Artery Dilation

Often PH is discovered incidentally when the pulmonary arteries are dilated. The Framingham Heart Study found that the 90th percentile for main pulmonary artery (MPA) size on noncontrast thoracic CT is 29 mm in males and 27 mm in females.[17] When the ratio of the MPA to the ascending aorta at the level of the bifurcation of the right pulmonary artery was measured, the 90th percentile for MPA-to-ascending aorta ratio was 0.91. Studies show that MPA diameter ≥ 29 mm is predictive of PH with sensitivity, specificity, positive predictive value, and negative predictive value of 87% to 88%, 42% to 89%, 70% to 97%, and 70%, respectively.[18,19] To avoid overdiagnosis of PH, some groups advocate a higher size threshold to raise the concern for PH. One study found that a threshold of MPA diameter greater than 29.5 mm was 71% sensitive and 79% specific for PH while raising the threshold to 31.5 mm increased the specificity to 90% at the cost of a sensitivity of 52%.[20] An improved specificity can reduce the need for further invasive testing to workup for PH.

Pulmonary Artery Filling Defects

Pulmonary artery filling defects, most commonly pulmonary embolism, can cause elevation of pulmonary artery pressures. Acute elevation of pulmonary artery pressure results in dilation of the main pulmonary artery, offering insight into the hemodynamic significance of the filling defect (**Fig. 2**). Chronic pulmonary artery mechanical obstruction leading to PH is quite rare. Causes of WHO Group 4 PH include flow obstruction due to chronic thromboembolic PH (discussed in a separate article in this issue) and, rarely, neoplasms such as pulmonary artery intimal sarcoma (**Fig. 3**).

PULMONARY FINDINGS
Ill-Defined Centrilobular Ground-Glass Nodules

Several patterns of lung nodules can occur in the setting of PH. One of the more common patterns is poorly-defined centrilobular ground-glass nodules (**Fig. 4**). These nodules often present in patients with longstanding, severe PH. Some studies have shown that in the setting of PH, these nodules represent cholesterol granulomas.[21]

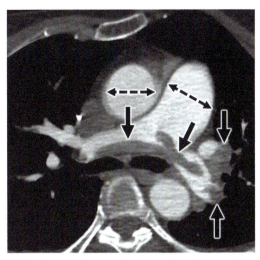

Fig. 2. Acute pulmonary hypertension due to pulmonary embolism. A computed tomography (CT) scan of a 69-year-old woman with coagulopathy and worsening shortness of breath shows multiple large filling defects (*arrows*) in the pulmonary arteries including a large saddle embolus resulting in dilation of the main pulmonary artery relative to the ascending aorta (*dashed arrows*).

Discrete centrilobular ground-glass nodules

Conversely, the presence of discrete centrilobular ground-glass nodules with well-defined margins can occur with pulmonary capillary hemangiomatosis (PCH). The distribution of centrilobular ground-glass nodules in PCH is diffuse and uniform (**Fig. 5**). The ground-glass nodules in PCH represent abnormal proliferation of pulmonary capillaries in the alveolar septa with associated alveolar hemorrhage.[22,23] While well-defined centrilobular pulmonary nodules are a hallmark of PCH, the imaging features of hypersensitivity pneumonitis (HP) are similar and can also present with PH. However, the clinical presentations are usually distinct.

Discrete Centrilobular Tree-In-Bud Nodules

Discrete tree-in-bud nodules are a rare manifestation of pulmonary tumor thrombotic microangiopathy resulting in PH.[24,25] This condition occurs in patients with malignancy that has metastasized hematogenously, resulting in occlusion of the pulmonary microvasculature as well as fibrointimal proliferation of the pulmonary arterioles, capillaries, and venules.[26]

Interlobular Septal Thickening and Confluent Ground-Glass Opacity

In the setting of PH, the presence of interlobular septal thickening and confluent ground-glass opacity raises the possibility of 2 main underlying causes. The most common cause is pulmonary edema due to congestive left heart failure (WHO Group 2 PH). Less commonly, this appearance represents pulmonary veno-occlusive disease (PVOD), a disease whereby the small pulmonary venules become progressively obstructed. Because the clinical presentation with heart failure and PVOD overlap, cardiac functional assessment, including echocardiography, will reveal normal cardiac function and right heart catheterization will show precapillary PH in the setting of PVOD[6,27] (**Fig. 6**). Further distinction between pulmonary arterial hypertension (PAH) and PVOD is achieved by administering vasodilators. Patients with

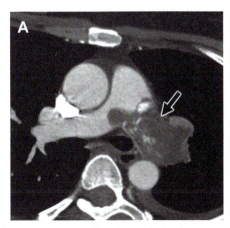 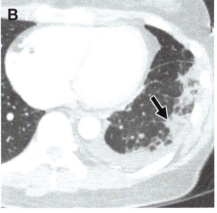

Fig. 3. Pulmonary hypertension due to intimal sarcoma. A CT scan of a 47-year-old woman with chest pain. (*A*) Large, occlusive soft tissue attenuation filling defect with internal osteoid matrix mineralization and rounded margins occupies the left pulmonary artery (*arrow*). (*B*) Peripheral wedge-shaped consolidation with areas of scarring (the latter not shown) suggests infarcts of varying ages suggesting that the aforementioned filling defect represents a chronic process.

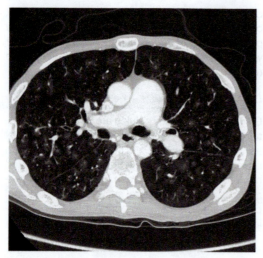

Fig. 4. Cholesterol granulomas manifesting as ill-defined centrilobular ground-glass nodules. A CT scan of a 37-year-old man with non-small cell lung cancer. Numerous ill-defined centrilobular ground-glass nodules in the presence of a dilated main pulmonary artery remained unchanged on multiple scans, a characteristic appearance suggestive of pulmonary hypertension.

PVOD typically experience clinical deterioration following administration of vasodilators, whereas patients with PAH typically exhibit improved blood flow and oxygenation.

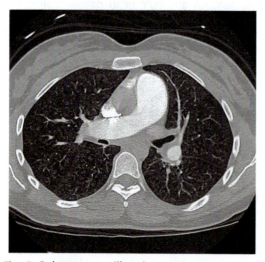

Fig. 5. Pulmonary capillary hemangiomatosis. A CT scan of a 30-year-old woman undergoing workup for pulmonary hypertension shows diffuse, uniform, discrete centrilobular ground-glass nodules with a dilated pulmonary artery, raising suspicion of pulmonary capillary hemangiomatosis. The patient had no symptoms of viral bronchiolitis and had no exposures to suggest hypersensitivity pneumonitis, both of which can sometimes have a similar appearance.

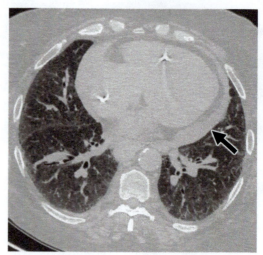

Fig. 6. Pulmonary veno-occlusive disease. A CT scan of a 55-year-old woman undergoing workup for pulmonary hypertension shows bilateral ground-glass opacities, septal thickening, and pericardial effusion. There was low suspicion for pulmonary edema with normal left ventricular function on a recent echocardiogram, raising suspicion of pulmonary veno-occlusive disease.

Pulmonary Fibrosis

Pulmonary fibrosis may be detected on CT performed as part of the evaluation for PH. Findings include reticulation, architectural distortion, traction bronchiectasis, honeycombing, mosaic perfusion, and air trapping (**Fig. 7**). PH is present in a greater proportion of patients who have more advanced pulmonary fibrosis.[28] Patients with PH and pulmonary fibrosis have a worse prognosis than those with PH caused by other entities.[29,30] Furthermore, patients with idiopathic pulmonary fibrosis (IPF) have a worse prognosis than those with connective tissue disease.[31] The increased morbidity and mortality of patients with advanced IPF and PH may be due to the increased risk of acute exacerbation compared to those without PH.[32] In patients with HP, PH is found more often in the fibrotic subtype.[33]

Pulmonary Cysts

Several cystic lung diseases are associated with development of PH.[34,35] For example, pulmonary Langerhans cell histiocytosis is a disorder associated predominantly with male smokers and produces upper lobe predominant nodules cysts with irregular contour. Also, lymphangioleiomyomatosis, a condition characterized by round, thin-walled cysts that are uniformly distributed throughout the lungs, is also associated with PH.

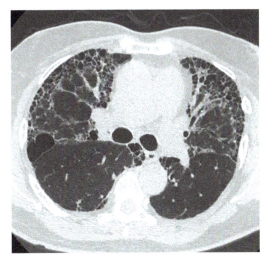

Fig. 7. Pulmonary hypertension due to chronic lung disease. A CT scan of a 73-year-old man with rheumatoid arthritis shows a dilated main pulmonary artery, a not uncommon finding in patients with various forms of pulmonary fibrosis.

Emphysema

Emphysema is present on CT in many patients with COPD. While centrilobular emphysema is the most common type, paraseptal and panlobular emphysema are also common subtypes (**Fig. 8**). Other findings associated with COPD include bronchial wall thickening, narrowing of the upper thoracic trachea in the coronal plane, and air trapping. Overall, about 40% of patients with COPD have PH, and the prevalence of PH in the COPD population increases with COPD severity.[36] Some patients with severe emphysema may undergo lung volume reduction surgery to remove the "dead-space" of the lung, which has been shown to improve PH.[37] An alternative technique to resection is less invasive endobronchial valve placement, which has also been shown in a small study to marginally improve pulmonary artery pressure

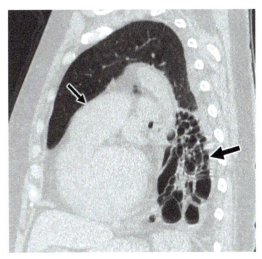

Fig. 9. Pulmonary hypertension due to bronchiectasis. A CT scan of a 68-year-old woman with severe left lower lobe bronchiectasis (*thick arrow*) shows dilation of the main pulmonary artery (*thin arrow*).

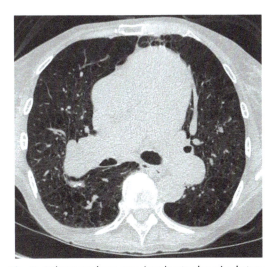

Fig. 8. Pulmonary hypertension due to chronic obstructive pulmonary disease (COPD). A CT scan of a 71-year-old woman shows severe emphysema and dilation of the central pulmonary arteries, the latter suggested on this image by the enlarged hilar vascular pedicles.

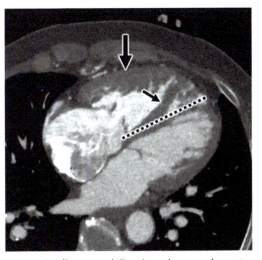

Fig. 10. Cardiac remodeling in pulmonary hypertension. A CT scan of a 68-year-old woman with pulmonary hypertension shows flattening of the interventricular septum (*dashed line*) and thickening of right ventricular structures such as the free wall (*thick arrow*) and moderator band (*thin arrow*). The right atrium and ventricle are also relatively dilated compared to the left heart chambers.

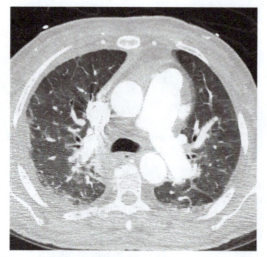

Fig. 11. Pulmonary hypertension due to left heart failure. A CT scan of a 58-year-old woman with ischemic cardiomyopathy and depressed left ventricle systolic function shows a mildly dilated main pulmonary artery and bilateral ground-glass opacities with bronchial wall and septal thickening. While such an appearance can be seen with pulmonary veno-occlusive disease, the CT findings are attributable to cardiogenic pulmonary edema given the history and commonality of this entity relative to the much rarer pulmonary veno-occlusive disease. In this case, CT findings resolved after appropriate management of heart disease.

can produce PH due to hypoxic vasoconstriction (Fig. 9). Of note, PH (measured via pulmonary artery dilation on CT) has been shown to be a predictor of mortality in patients with bronchiectasis with a hazard ratio of 1.24.[39]

CARDIAC FINDINGS
Right Heart Morphology

PH can cause structural changes of the right heart as elevated pressure in the pulmonary arteries is transmitted to the right ventricle, resulting in right ventricular dilation and flattening or leftward bowing of the interventricular septum, notably during ventricular systole (Fig. 10). If the elevated right ventricular pressures are long-standing, right ventricular hypertrophy can develop. When the right atrium is also affected by elevated pressures, the right atrium can dilate, which is associated with a poorer prognosis.[40]

Left Heart Morphology

Left heart disease can be a cause of PH. Any cause of left ventricular failure, in the setting of ischemic or nonischemic cardiomyopathy, can lead to pulmonary venous and arterial hypertension. Causes of ischemic cardiomyopathy include myocardial infarct from coronary artery atherosclerosis, coronary artery dissection, or embolism to the coronary arteries (Fig. 11). Causes of nonischemic cardiomyopathy include genetic or toxin-mediated etiologies, diabetes, arrhythmia, and valvular disease.

immediately and 3 months following endobronchial valve placement.[38]

Bronchiectasis

Bronchiectasis from chronic infectious or inflammatory disorders such as cystic fibrosis or chronic nontuberculous mycobacterial infection

Cardiovascular Shunts and Congenital Heart Disease

Congenital cardiovascular shunts, if uncorrected, can lead to PH. Chronic left-to-right shunting

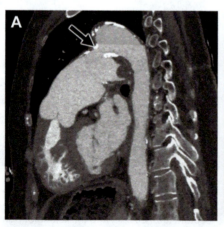
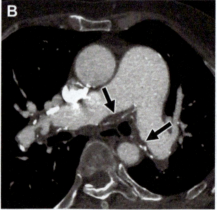

Fig. 12. Pulmonary hypertension due to cardiovascular shunt. (A) A CT scan of a 68-year-old woman shows a large, calcified patent ductus arteriosus (arrow) and dilated main pulmonary artery. (B) Due to the longstanding severe volume and ensuing pressure overload, the patient developed atherosclerotic plaques with intimal calcifications of the pulmonary arteries (arrows).

introduces an excess volume of blood into the pulmonary circulation, leading to remodeling of the pulmonary vascular bed. Shunts may take the form of atrial or ventricular septal defects, patent ductus arteriosus, or partial anomalous pulmonary venous return. While echocardiography can help detect the presence of atrial and ventricular septal defects, CT and MR imaging offer a more comprehensive evaluation for extracardiac shunts, which may not be well characterized on echocardiography, particularly in older children and adults (**Fig. 12**). Eventually, long-standing uncorrected shunts result in severe PH with suprasystemic right heart pressures, resulting in reversal of flow across the shunt and Eisenmenger syndrome (**Fig. 13**). Beyond simple shunts, CT and MR imaging are helpful in evaluating the potential underlying sources of PH in patients with complex congenital heart disease. Both modalities offer noninvasive morphologic characterization of the cardiovascular system and enable assessment for precapillary and/or post-capillary sources of PH such as segmental pulmonary artery stenosis or pulmonary vein obstruction (**Fig. 14**). CT with retrospective electrocardiogram-gating and MR imaging also offer the ability to measure cardiac chamber volumes and ventricular function. Furthermore, cardiac MR imaging can identify and quantify valvular stenosis or regurgitation. Of note, in patients with complex congenital heart disease, cross-sectional imaging is used in combination with echocardiography and cardiac catheterization is used to identify, characterize, and manage PH.

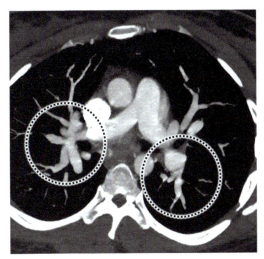

Fig. 14. Congenital segmental pulmonary artery stenosis. A CT scan of a 35-year-old woman with congenital heart disease and pulmonary hypertension shows alternating stenosis and dilation of several bilateral segmental pulmonary arteries, which likely contributed to elevation of main pulmonary artery pressure.

MEDIASTINAL FINDINGS
Mediastinal Lymphadenopathy

Enlargement of mediastinal nodes can occur in patients with PH and may be reactive in the setting of

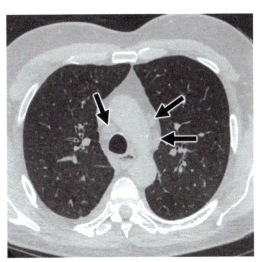

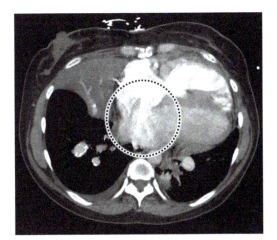

Fig. 13. Eisenmenger syndrome. A Computed tomography angiography (CTA) scan during pulmonary artery phase of a 46-year-old woman with uncorrected atrial septal defect shows dense contrast crossing from the right atrium to the left atrium across the interatrial septum (*dashed circle*). This reversal of flow suggests suprasystemic pressures in the right heart chambers relative to the left.

Fig. 15. Mediastinal lymphadenopathy in a patient with pulmonary hypertension. A CT scan of a 58-year-old man undergoing workup of pulmonary hypertension with normal cardiac function as assessed by echocardiogram shows multi-station mediastinal lymphadenopathy (*arrows*) with concomitant findings of bilateral ground-glass opacities, bronchial wall thickening, and septal thickening, Given the normal left ventricular function and presence of lymphadenopathy, these findings raise suspicion for pulmonary veno-occlusive disease.

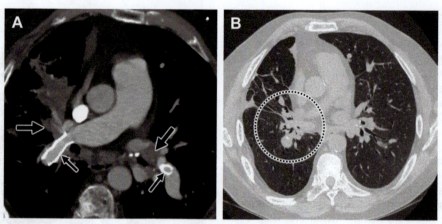

Fig. 16. Pulmonary hypertension due to fibrosing mediastinitis. (*A*) A CT scan of a 68-year-old man with previous histoplasmosis shows bilateral hilar soft tissue (*thick arrows*) with fine calcifications. Due to stenosis of the pulmonary arteries caused by mediastinal fibrosis, stents were placed (*thin arrows*). (*B*) Stenosis of other structures including the bronchi can occur as in this case, helping increase diagnostic confidence.

ILD and PCH/PVOD or granuloma laden in the setting of sarcoidosis (**Fig. 15**).[41] Of interest, a histologic study suggested that the underlying cause of mediastinal lymphadenopathy in patients with PVOD and PCH may be venous congestion and altered venolymphatic flow.[41]

Mediastinal Soft Tissue and Vascular Stenosis

When there is chronic mediastinal lymphadenopathy and granulomatous inflammation, fibrosing mediastinitis can occur, often from infection with *Histoplasma capsulatum* (**Fig. 16**). Other conditions that present with extensive mediastinal lymphadenopathy include sarcoidosis and IgG4 sclerosing disease. This extensive lymphadenopathy may eventually result in vascular and/or airway stenosis. While the central veins such as the superior vena cava are more commonly narrowed, the pulmonary arteries or veins can also be affected, resulting in PH.[42–44]

ABDOMINAL FINDINGS

The upper abdomen is often included on chest and cardiac CT and MR imaging. Signs of PH described in the echocardiography literature include distension and impaired collapsibility of the upper inferior vena cava (IVC).[45] Distension of the IVC and hepatic veins may also be observed on CT and MR imaging. Conversely, the cause of PH may be secondary to an abdominal process. Portopulmonary hypertension is common in the setting of hepatic cirrhosis. When the typical features of cirrhosis are present, including a nodular hepatic contour, portal and splenic vein dilation, upper abdominal and paraesophageal varices, and splenomegaly, it is prudent to inspect the chest for signs of PH (**Fig. 17**).[46,47]

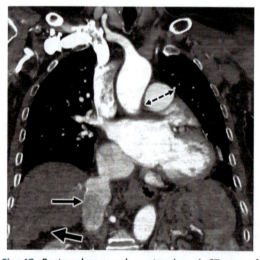

Fig. 17. Portopulmonary hypertension. A CT scan of a 75-year-old man with hepatic cirrhosis shows a mildly dilated main pulmonary artery (*dashed double-head arrow*) and nodular hepatic contour (*arrow*). The upper inferior vena cava is also dilated (*thin arrow*), not uncommon in patients with pulmonary hypertension.

SUMMARY

PH is uncommon but presents a significant problem with poor outcome if untreated. The diagnostic evaluation for PH is aimed at revealing the underlying cause, which most commonly are left heart disease, chronic lung disease, and idiopathic PH. Unfortunately, patients may have more than 1 cause of PH, necessitating several forms of testing including echocardiography, right heart catheterization, and chest CT. Understanding the role of radiologic imaging in the diagnosis of PH is important as it allows the radiologist to contribute vital information to the care of PH patients in the multidisciplinary setting.

CLINICS CARE POINTS

- Pulmonary hypertension is defined as a mean pulmonary artery pressure of ≥20 mmHg.
- Left heart disease and chronic lung disease constitute the top two causes of pulmonary hypertension and the early stage of diagnostic workup often involves echocardiography and thoracic CT to evaluate the heart and lungs.
- Main pulmonary artery size ≥29 mm offers relatively high sensitivity in detecting pulmonary hypertension, though higher thresholds such as ~32 mm offer higher specificity.
- Thoracic CT helps include and exclude both pulmonary and primary vascular causes of pulmonary hypertension.
- Some conditions, such as pulmonary edema from heart failure and pulmonary venoocclusive disease, can appear indistinguishable; however, other clinical data such as echocardiography and right heart catheterization results can prove useful in arriving at the most likely underlying etiology of the imaging appearance.

DISCLOSURE

The authors have no relevant financial disclosures related to the contents of this paper.

REFERENCES

1. Wijeratne DT, Lajkosz K, Brogly SB, et al. Increasing incidence and prevalence of World Health Organization Groups 1 to 4 Pulmonary Hypertension: A Population-Based Cohort Study in Ontario, Canada. Circ Cardiovasc Qual Outcomes 2018;11(2):e003973.
2. Kovacs G, Berghold A, Scheidl S, et al. Pulmonary arterial pressure during rest and exercise in healthy subjects: a systematic review. Eur Respir J 2009;34(4):888–94.
3. Galiè N, Humbert M, Vachiery JL, et al. 2015 ESC/ERS Guidelines for the diagnosis and treatment of pulmonary hypertension: The Joint Task Force for the Diagnosis and Treatment of Pulmonary Hypertension of the European Society of Cardiology (ESC) and the European Respiratory Society (ERS): Endorsed by: Association for European Paediatric and Congenital Cardiology (AEPC), International Society for Heart and Lung Transplantation (ISHLT). Eur Heart J 2016;37(1):67–119.
4. Hoeper MM, Bogaard HJ, Condliffe R, et al. Definitions and diagnosis of pulmonary hypertension. J Am Coll Cardiol 2013;62(25 Suppl):D42–50.
5. Heresi GA, Minai OA, Tonelli AR, et al. Clinical characterization and survival of patients with borderline elevation in pulmonary artery pressure. Pulm Circ 2013;3(4):916–25.
6. Humbert M, Kovacs G, Hoeper MM, et al. ESC/ERS Guidelines for the diagnosis and treatment of pulmonary hypertension. Eur Heart J 2022;43(38):3618–731.
7. Simonneau G, Hoeper MM. The revised definition of pulmonary hypertension: exploring the impact on patient management. Eur Heart J Suppl 2019;21(Suppl K):K4–8.
8. Frost A, Badesch D, Gibbs JSR, et al. Diagnosis of pulmonary hypertension. Eur Respir J 2019;53(1):1801904.
9. Rich JD, Rich S. Clinical diagnosis of pulmonary hypertension. Circulation 2014;130(20):1820–30.
10. Brown LM, Chen H, Halpern S, et al. Delay in recognition of pulmonary arterial hypertension: factors identified from the REVEAL Registry. Chest 2011;140(1):19–26.
11. Farmakis IT, Demerouti E, Karyofyllis P, et al. Echocardiography in pulmonary arterial hypertension: is it time to reconsider its prognostic utility? J Clin Med 2021;10(13):2826.
12. Topyła-Putowska W, Tomaszewski M, Wysokiński A, et al. Echocardiography in pulmonary arterial hypertension: comprehensive evaluation and technical considerations. J Clin Med 2021;10(15):3229.
13. Broncano J, Bhalla S, Gutierrez FR, et al. Cardiac MRI in pulmonary hypertension: from magnet to bedside. Radiographics 2020;40(4):982–1002.
14. Chaouat A, Bugnet AS, Kadaoui N, et al. Severe pulmonary hypertension and chronic obstructive pulmonary disease. Am J Respir Crit Care Med 2005;172(2):189–94.
15. Kimura M, Taniguchi H, Kondoh Y, et al. Pulmonary hypertension as a prognostic indicator at the initial evaluation in idiopathic pulmonary fibrosis. Respiration 2013;85(6):456–63.
16. Shorr AF, Helman DL, Davies DB, et al. Pulmonary hypertension in advanced sarcoidosis: epidemiology and clinical characteristics. Eur Respir J 2005;25(5):783–8.
17. Truong QA, Massaro JM, Rogers IS, et al. Reference values for normal pulmonary artery dimensions by noncontrast cardiac computed tomography: the Framingham Heart Study. Circ Cardiovasc Imaging 2012;5(1):147–54.

18. Tan RT, Kuzo R, Goodman LR, et al. Utility of CT scan evaluation for predicting pulmonary hypertension in patients with parenchymal lung disease. Medical College of Wisconsin Lung Transplant Group. Chest 1998;113(5):1250–6.
19. Ratanawatkul P, Oh A, Richards JC, et al. Performance of pulmonary artery dimensions measured on high-resolution computed tomography scan for identifying pulmonary hypertension. ERJ Open Res 2020;6(1):00232–2019.
20. Mahammedi A, Oshmyansky A, Hassoun PM, et al. Pulmonary artery measurements in pulmonary hypertension: the role of computed tomography. J Thorac Imag 2013;28(2):96–103.
21. Nolan RL, McAdams HP, Sporn TA, et al. Pulmonary cholesterol granulomas in patients with pulmonary artery hypertension: chest radiographic and CT findings. AJR Am J Roentgenol 1999;172(5):1317–9.
22. Weatherald J, Dorfmüller P, Perros F, et al. Pulmonary capillary haemangiomatosis: a distinct entity? Eur Respir Rev 2020;29(156):190168.
23. Guzman S, Khan MS, Chodakiewitz Y, et al. Pulmonary capillary hemangiomatosis: a lesson learned. Autops Case Rep 2019;9(3):e2019111.
24. Franquet T, Giménez A, Prats R, et al. Thrombotic microangiopathy of pulmonary tumors: a vascular cause of tree-in-bud pattern on CT. AJR Am J Roentgenol 2002;179(4):897–9.
25. Price LC, Seckl MJ, Dorfmüller P, et al. Tumoral pulmonary hypertension. Eur Respir Rev 2019;28(151):180065.
26. Kumar N, Price LC, Montero MA, et al. Pulmonary tumour thrombotic microangiopathy: unclassifiable pulmonary hypertension? Eur Respir J 2015;46(4):1214–7.
27. Montani D, Lau EM, Dorfmüller P, et al. Pulmonary veno-occlusive disease. Eur Respir J 2016;47(5):1518–34.
28. Kacprzak A, Tomkowski W, Szturmowicz M. Pulmonary hypertension in the course of interstitial lung diseases-a personalised approach is needed to identify a dominant cause and provide an effective therapy. Diagnostics 2023;13(14):2354.
29. Chebib N, Mornex JF, Traclet J, et al. Pulmonary hypertension in chronic lung diseases: comparison to other pulmonary hypertension groups. Pulm Circ 2018;8(2). 2045894018775056.
30. Gall H, Felix JF, Schneck FK, et al. The giessen pulmonary hypertension registry: survival in pulmonary hypertension subgroups. J Heart Lung Transplant 2017;36(9):957–67.
31. Alhamad EH, Cal JG, Alrajhi NN, et al. Predictors of mortality in patients with interstitial lung disease-associated pulmonary hypertension. J Clin Med 2020;9(12):3828.
32. Judge EP, Fabre A, Adamali HI, et al. Acute exacerbations and pulmonary hypertension in advanced idiopathic pulmonary fibrosis. Eur Respir J 2012;40(1):93–100.
33. Trushenko NV, Suvorova OA, Nekludova GV, et al. Predictors of pulmonary hypertension and right ventricular dysfunction in patients with hypersensitivity pneumonitis. Life (Basel) 2023;13(6):1348.
34. Le Pavec J, Lorillon G, Jaïs X, et al. Pulmonary Langerhans cell histiocytosis-associated pulmonary hypertension: clinical characteristics and impact of pulmonary arterial hypertension therapies. Chest 2012;142(5):1150–7.
35. Freitas CSG, Baldi BG, Jardim C, et al. Pulmonary hypertension in lymphangioleiomyomatosis: prevalence, severity and the role of carbon monoxide diffusion capacity as a screening method. Orphanet J Rare Dis 2017;12(1):74.
36. Zhang L, Liu Y, Zhao S, et al. The incidence and prevalence of pulmonary hypertension in the COPD population: a systematic review and meta-analysis. Int J Chronic Obstr Pulm Dis 2022;17:1365–79.
37. Akil A, Ziegeler S, Rehers S, et al. Lung volume reduction surgery reduces pulmonary arterial hypertension associated with severe lung emphysema and hypercapnia. ASAIO J 2023;69(2):218–24.
38. Eberhardt R, Gerovasili V, Kontogianni K, et al. Endoscopic lung volume reduction with endobronchial valves in patients with severe emphysema and established pulmonary hypertension. Respiration 2015;89(1):41–8.
39. Devaraj A, Wells AU, Meister MG, et al. Pulmonary hypertension in patients with bronchiectasis: prognostic significance of CT signs. AJR Am J Roentgenol 2011;196(6):1300–4.
40. D'Alonzo GE, Barst RJ, Ayres SM, et al. Survival in patients with primary pulmonary hypertension. Results from a national prospective registry. Ann Intern Med 1991;115(5):343–9.
41. Thomas de Montpréville V, Dulmet E, Fadel E, et al. Lymph node pathology in pulmonary veno-occlusive disease and pulmonary capillary heamangiomatosis. Virchows Arch 2008;453(2):171–6.
42. Gustafson MR, Moulton MJ. Fibrosing mediastinitis with severe bilateral pulmonary artery narrowing: RV-RPA bypass with a homograft conduit. Tex Heart Inst J 2012;39(3):412–5.
43. Argueta F, Villafuerte D, Castaneda-Nerio J, et al. Successful management of fibrosing mediastinitis with severe vascular compromise: Report of two cases and literature review. Respir Med Case Rep 2020;29:100987.
44. Ye JR, Hu SY, Lin YH, et al. Surgery for fibrosing mediastinitis with severe pulmonary hypertension due to pulmonary venous stenosis. J Heart Lung Transplant 2024;43(1):28–31.

45. Habib G, Torbicki A. The role of echocardiography in the diagnosis and management of patients with pulmonary hypertension. Eur Respir Rev 2010;19(118): 288–99.
46. Devaraj A, Loveridge R, Bosanac D, et al. Portopulmonary hypertension: improved detection using CT and echocardiography in combination. Eur Radiol 2014;24(10):2385–93.
47. Hayashi H, Oda S, Kidoh M, et al. Pulmonary arterial hypertension associated with portal hypertension: Noninvasive comprehensive assessment using computed tomography. Radiol Case Rep 2024;19(2):671–4.

Imaging of Acute Pulmonary Embolism
An Update

Kiran Batra, MD[a,b,]*, Fernando U. Kay, MD, PhD[a], Robert C. Sibley, MD[a], Ronald M. Peshock, MD[a,b]

KEYWORDS

- Pulmonary embolism • Artificial intelligence • Update • Dual-energy CT (DECT) • Artifact • Triage

KEY POINTS

- Imaging is essential in the evaluation and management of acute pulmonary embolism.
- Advances in multi-energy CT including dual-energy CT and photon-counting CT have allowed faster scans with lower radiation dose and optimal image quality.
- Artificial intelligence has a potential role in triaging potentially positive examinations and could serve as a second reader.

INTRODUCTION

The annual incidence of acute pulmonary embolism (PE) is one in 1000 person worldwide.[1] PE accounts for 100,000 deaths annually in the United States.[2] Although the true mortality rate from undiagnosed PE is low, the diagnosis itself can be debilitating as recovery from acute PE encompasses complications like bleeding secondary to anticoagulation treatment, recurrent venous thromboembolism, chronic thromboembolic pulmonary hypertension, and prolonged psychological stress.[3] Post-pulmonary-embolism syndrome refers to the functional and exercise limitations 1 year after a diagnosis of PE and occurred in about 50% of patients in one cohort.[3,4] A timely and expert diagnosis of PE is therefore important.

PE usually occurs when a clot enters the pulmonary circulation, most commonly arising from deep calf veins. Imaging is crucial for appropriate diagnosis and management of acute PE. CT pulmonary angiography (CTPA) is the most common modality used in the evaluation of suspected acute PE with a reported sensitivity and specificity of 96% to 100% and 89% to 98%,[5] respectively.

Acute PE can be a challenging clinical diagnosis to make due to nonspecific presenting signs and symptoms, and about two-thirds of patients may be asymptomatic.[6] A number of clinical scoring systems like the Wells criteria, the Geneva score, and the Pulmonary Embolism Rule-out Criteria are used in combination with values like age adjusted D-dimer to determine the clinical risk of PE[7] (**Table 1**).

The recent technological advancements like dual-energy CT and emerging technology like photon-counting CT (PCCT) show promising results in improving the image quality of CTPA even with lower radiation dose. Artificial intelligence (AI) with robust deep learning algorithms has shown encouraging results as a potential second reader and as a triage tool for identifying potentially positive CTPA. The authors discuss the role of imaging including newer technologies and the potential roles for AI in acute PE.

IMAGING TECHNIQUES
Chest Radiography

Chest radiography has limited utility in the diagnosis of PE but is useful in excluding other causes of

---

[a] Department of Radiology, University of Texas Southwestern Medical Center, Dallas, TX 75390, USA; [b] Department of Internal Medicine, University of Texas Southwestern Medical Center, Dallas, TX 75390, USA
* Corresponding author.
E-mail address: kiran.batra@utsouthwestern.edu

Table 1
Clinical scoring systems used in combination with D-Dimer values to show the clinical risk of pulmonary embolism

Wells Score		Geneva Score			PERC Score
Criteria	Points	Criteria	Revised Pts	Simplified Pts	Criteria
PE most likely diagnosis	3.0	Age >65 y	1.0	1.0	Age ≥50 y
Signs and symptoms of DVT	3.0	Previous DVT or PE	3.0	1.0	HR ≥100 bpm
HR >100 bpm	1.5	Surgery/fracture within 1 mo	2.0	1.0	SPO_2 <95% while patient is breathing room air
Immobilization for >3 days/surgery in the previous 4 wk	1.5	Active cancer	2.0	1.0	Swelling in one leg
Previous DVT or PE	1.5	Pain in one lower limb	3.0	1.0	Hemoptysis
Hemoptysis	1.0	Hemoptysis	2.0	1.0	Surgery/trauma in the last 4 wk
Active cancer	1.0	HR between 75 and 94 BPM	3.0	1.0	
		Heart rate ≥95 BPM	5.0	2.0	Previous DVT or PE
		Pain on lower limb deep-vein palpitation and edema in one leg	4.0	1.0	Hormone use

Abbreviations: BPM: beats per minute; DVT, deep venous thrombus; HR, heart rate; PE, pulmonary embolism; Pts, points; SPO2, peripheral Oxygen saturation.

acute chest pain and dyspnea such as pulmonary edema, pneumonia, or pneumothorax. Rarely encountered indirect signs that may indicate acute PE include the Fleischer sign (an enlarged main pulmonary artery secondary to the embolus and acute pulmonary hypertension), Palla's sign (an enlarged right descending pulmonary artery before a vascular occlusion in acute PE), and the Westermark sign (acute cut-off of the pulmonary artery with regional hypo perfusion). PE can lead to pulmonary infarction, manifesting as a subpleural wedge shaped opacity with apex directed toward the hilum (Hampton hump; **Fig. 1**A–C), but this sign has a low sensitivity (22%) and intermediate specificity (82%). Other nonspecific findings include atelectasis, pleural effusion, elevated hemidiaphragm, and vascular redistribution with sensitivity of 10% to 36% and specificity of 70% to 85%.[8]

CT Pulmonary Angiography

CTPA is the diagnostic imaging test of choice for the evaluation of patients with suspected acute PE as it is widely available, fast, minimally invasive, and cost-effective.

CTPA has undergone remarkable advancements over years.[9] The transition from single to multi-detector CT (MDCT) technology significantly allowed improvement in spatial and temporal resolution, acquisition speed, and overall diagnostic accuracy.[10] A meta-analysis of state-of-the-art MDCT, including 16 studies with 4,392 participants, showed pooled sensitivity and specificity estimates of 94% and 98%, respectively.[11]

Further advancements in scanning technology have continued to refine the role of CTPA in acute PE diagnosis. The introduction of dual-source scanners has been particularly notable, enabling high helical pitch scanning and spectral scanning. High-pitch scanning offers the potential to reduce both contrast and radiation doses while maintaining sufficient image quality for accurate diagnosis.[12] For example, a recent study showed that high-pitch CTPA using a contrast dose as small as 20 mL, compared to the standard 50 mL, resulted in diagnostic images for detecting acute PE and significantly reduced radiation exposure in patients without obesity.[13]

Additionally, a study comparing high-pitch CT scans to standard pitch protocols found that the former significantly improved quality of the scan, from decrease in motion artifacts[14] thereby, allowing optimal evaluation of cardiac structures. The mean effective dose was also significantly lower for high-pitch scans, while maintaining comparable image quality in terms of pulmonary vessel attenuation, signal-to-noise ratio, and contrast-to-noise ratio (CNR).[12]

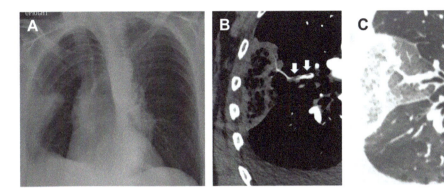

Fig. 1. (A) A 52 year old man with acute chest pain. Frontal chest radiograph shows a wedge-shaped opacity in the periphery of the right lung suggestive of an infarction (Hampton hump). (B) 52 year old man with acute chest pain axial CTPA shows a nonocclusive filling defect in the enlarged anterior segmental branch (arrows) in the right lower lobe consistent with an acute embolus. Peripheral consolidation corresponds to the abnormality on the radiograph. Note small right pleural effusion (C) 52 year old man with acute chest pain axial CTPA (lung window settings) shows a reverse halo sign, corresponding to a pulmonary infarct.

The pulmonary arteries need to be adequately opacified so that the thrombus is distinguished from intraluminal contrast material. A theoretic minimum of 93 Hounsfield (HU) intraluminal density is required for the detection of acute PE and of 211 HU to detect chronic embolus.[15] Optimal timing for intravenous contrast bolus can be determined using bolus tracking, timing bolus, and empirical techniques. A saline injection of the same volume is administered after contrast to reduce the dense streak artifacts from undiluted contrast in the superior vena cava (SVC). The exact contrast material volume, concentration, and injection rate depend on the scanner characteristics.

Signs of acute PE on CT are based on if the PE is acute or chronic and occlusive or nonocclusive. Total non-opacification of the vessel occurs from occlusion. A "polo mint" sign (**Fig. 2**) implies a central well-defined filling defect surrounded by contrast when oriented perpendicular to the long axis of the vessel. The "railway "sign (**Fig. 3**) refers to the linear filling defect in the vessel when the orientation of the vessel is parallel to its long axis. A saddle embolus occurs when the thrombus branches across the main pulmonary artery bifurcation and into the main branch vessels (**Fig. 4**).[9] A nonocclusive filling defect can also present as an eccentric clot, but typically, the vessel is enlarged, and the filling defect makes an acute angle with the wall (**Fig. 5**), unlike in chronic embolus where the involved vessel is attenuated, and the filling defect is concave and aligns at an obtuse angle.

Detection of acute embolus in the subsegmental vessels, which affects the fourth division and further distal pulmonary arterial branches, became possible with the advent of multidetector row CTPA.[16] The detection rate of subsegmental has increased with multidetector CT and ranges from 3% to 12%, but the significance of their detection in a low-risk patient without deep venous thrombosis is controversial.[17]

On CTPA, a pulmonary infarct appears as a peripheral wedge-shaped focus of non-enhancing consolidation intermixed with ground-glass opacity (GGO). A "reverse-halo" or "atoll" (see **Fig. 1**) appearance consisting of central GGO surrounded by a complete or incomplete rim of consolidation is an occasional finding. The central GGO usually represents coagulative necrosis. Although there are quantitative scoring systems to assess clot burden and obstruction index in the pulmonary vessels, use in clinical workflow is not routine.[18,19]

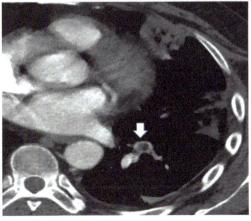

Fig. 2. A 52 year old man with acute dyspnea. Axial CTPA orthogonal to an expanded left lower lobe lateral segmental pulmonary artery shows a "polo mint" sign of acute PE (arrow). Note the peripheral opacities in the lingual consistent with infarcts.

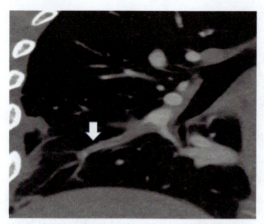

Fig. 3. A 30 year old woman with sickle cell disease presenting with daily fevers and pleuritic chest pain. Coronal reformatted CTPA (bone window settings) image shows a central filling defect in the right lower lobe superior and lateral segmental branches (*arrow*), surrounded by parallel contrast column consistent with "railway sign" compatible with a nonocclusive acute PE. Note the peripheral wedge-shaped opacity consistent with an infarct.

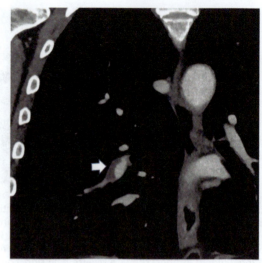

Fig. 5. A 61 year old man with renal cell cancer with acute chest pain and elevated D-dimer. Coronal CTPA image shows a low-attenuation nonocclusive eccentric acute pulmonary embolus in the right interlobar pulmonary artery with acute angle to the vessel wall (*arrow*).

Several risk stratification parameters can be derived from CTPA such as right ventricular strain and lung perfusion. Imaging features of right ventricular strain include an increased right-to-left ventricle ratio (>1.1) in the axial plane, contiguous reflux of contrast into the inferior vena cava (IVC) and hepatic veins and flattening of interventricular septum (**Fig. 6**A–B).[20] Several studies have correlated the right ventricle- left ventricle (RV-LV) ratio with 30 day mortality. In acute PE, an RV diameter of 53 mm or more and a CT obstruction index greater than 70% are associated with increased 30 day mortality in one retrospective single-center study.[21] A 4 chamber RV-LV ratio greater than 0.9 was associated with poor clinical outcome and increased risk of death within 30 days in combination with elevated high-sensitivity cardiac troponin-I in a retrospective study.[22] However, another study showed that RV/LV greater than 1 did not predict severe outcomes (odds ratio [OR] = 0.73, $P=0$).[23] Main PA diameter and interventricular septal bowing have an association with short-term adverse outcomes in patients with acute PE.[24,25]

Artifacts on CT Pulmonary Angiography

Motion artifacts from cardiac pulsation or patient movement and streak artifacts from undiluted contrast in the SVC can degrade image quality of CTPA. Suboptimal contrast enhancement can occur in CTPA examinations from underlying physiology like decreased cardiac output. The radiologist should be aware of these appearances and be able to distinguish artifacts from true contrast enhancement to avoid erroneous interpretation, especially in critically ill patients. Some of these artifacts are also described as "smoke-like" artifacts (**Fig. 7**A–C and **8**A–C) in vessels secondary to mixing of unopacified blood with contrast and more frequent in the modern scanners

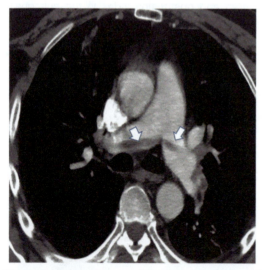

Fig. 4. A 48 year old man with acute chest pain and elevated D-dimer. Axial CTPA shows a low-attenuation embolus across the bifurcation of the pulmonary artery, consistent with a "saddle embolus" configuration (*arrows*).

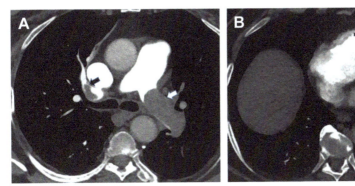

Fig. 6. (*A*) A 77 year old woman with acute chest discomfort. Axial CTPA shows near occlusive thrombus in the left main (*white arrow*) and nonocclusive clots (*black arrow*) in the right upper lobar pulmonary artery consistent with acute central PE. (*B*) A 77 year old woman with acute chest discomfort. Axial CTPA shows that the right ventricle is dilated suggestive of right ventricular strain.

secondary to increased temporal resolution and shorter scan time. Transient interruption of flow to contrast can occur if there is mixing of unopacified blood from the IVC with contrast coming from the SVC exacerbated by the Valsalva maneuver and culminating in poor opacification of the pulmonary vasculature.[26]

A true thrombus appears as a well-defined filling defect with sharp and convex margins. The mean attenuation of acute PE was at 33HU+-15 HU, in one study and, 90% of the emboli had an attenuation less than 100 HU.[27] Improper display of the window settings, particularly narrow window width (WW) and high window level (WL), can lead to accentuation of the heterogeneous attenuation of the "smoke-like" appearance. Window settings (WL-40/WW-400) based on the double-half method are a standard practice that should be adequate for identification of PE and reducing this artifact.[28]

Scanning very early can create artifacts at the leading edge of the contrast bolus and form an intravascular contrast level in pulmonary artery branches but typically, a straight interface with the dependent contrast medium allows identification as artifact. Regional alterations of pulmonary blood flow secondary to resistance in chronic parenchymal lung disease occur due to vasoconstriction from hypoxia (see **Figs. 7** and **8**). Narrowing of the vessel upstream in pulmonary venous stenosis or downstream due to narrowing of pulmonary artery in conditions like fibrosing mediastinitis creates slow flow mimicking emboli. Flow from venous collateral due to decreased cardiac output or bronchial artery collaterals (see **Fig. 8**) in bronchiectasis can also create filling defects, but the proximity to the bronchial collaterals should be a clue. The latter can be distinguished by acquiring the scan in the systemic arterial phase with saline flushes.[29]

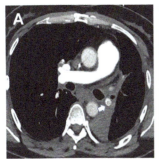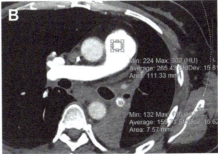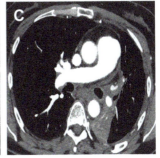

Fig. 7. (*A*) A 51 year old woman with shortness of breath and fever. Axial CTPA shows a filling defect (*arrow*) in the left lower interlobar pulmonary artery with ill-defined margins. Note atelectasis in the left lower lobe. (*B*) A 51 year old woman with shortness of breath and fever. The mean attenuation region of interest (ROI) of the filling defect is at 132 HU, higher than would be expected for an actual embolus. (*C*) A 51 year old woman with shortness of breath and fever axial CTPA after 12 hours arterial and venous (not shown) phase shows no filling defect confirming flow artifact secondary to downstream atelectasis and consolidation (not shown).

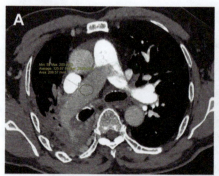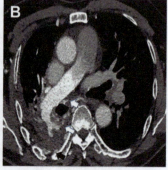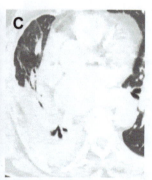

Fig. 8. (*A*) A 63 year old woman with pleuritic chest pain, elevated D-dimer, and history of treatment of necrotizing pneumonia. Axial CTPA shows heterogeneous nonopacification of the right main pulmonary artery, an ROI mean of 126 HU, and smoke-like filling defects in the main and left pulmonary artery. (*B*) A 63 year old woman with pleuritic chest pain, elevated D-dimer, and history of treatment of necrotizing pneumonia. Repeat CT chest with contrast injection timed off the descending aorta shows optimal filling of the right main pulmonary artery from extensive right intercostal, and bronchial collaterals (*arrows*). Note that the collateral and the aorta are similar in attenuation. (*C*) A 63 year old woman with pleuritic chest pain, elevated D-dimer, and history of treatment of necrotizing pneumonia. Axial chest CT (lung window settings) shows chronic consolidation/collapse with bronchiectasis following treatment of necrotizing pneumonia.

Flow artifacts can be managed by obtaining a delayed acquisition in a venous phase or by using the bolus triggering method with region of interest (ROI) on the descending aorta at 1 to 3 minutes or single-phase split bolus technique. The earlier acquisitions lead to improvement in contrast enhancement of the pulmonary vasculature and at the same time allow aortic pathologies to be excluded.[30]

Technical Advances on CTPA, Multi-energy CT, and Photon-counting CT

A significant advancement in CTPA entails introduction of MECT, initially enabled by dual-source scanners. This technology is supported by innovations, such as rapid kVp switching, dual-spin CT, split-beam CT, dual-layer CT, and PCCT.[31] MECT can provide low virtual monoenergetic (VMI) and iodine-based material decomposition images. Low VMI enhances the apparent CT numbers of iodine, thereby improving the CNR compared to low kVp imaging (**Fig. 9**) alone, potentially offering superior evaluation of vascular structures and enhanced detection of PE.[32,33]

Iodine-based material decomposition imaging has been adopted as a surrogate method for assessing perfusion.[34,35] MECT perfusion approximates perfusion at a single time point, unlike dynamic CT or MR perfusion, and depends on acquisition timing and hemodynamics. Pulmonary blood volume (PBV) images are derived by calculating the mean enhancement of the pulmonary parenchyma relative to a reference vessel (usually the pulmonary trunk) and correcting this ratio with a calibration factor.[36] PBV imaging has been effective in identifying perfusion defects related to pulmonary emboli (**Fig. 10**A, B), with reported per segment sensitivity and specificity of 83% and 99%, respectively, when compared to perfusion scintigraphy.[37] Another study indicated that iodine imaging showed a sensitivity and specificity of 77% and 98%, respectively, compared to single-photon emission computed tomography (SPECT)/CT.[38] Combining MECT iodine imaging with CT

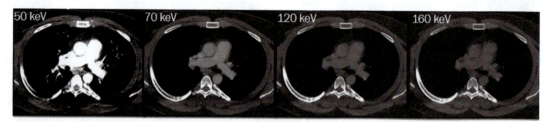

Fig. 9. A 45 year old man with dyspnea. Virtual monoenergetic imaging (VMI) improves vascular visualization in suboptimal CT pulmonary angiography. Note the limited opacification of the central pulmonary arteries as assessed on 70 keV images (ie, 120 kVp-equivalent images). CT numbers associated with the presence of iodine are enhanced at 50 keV VMI, allowing for improved image quality.

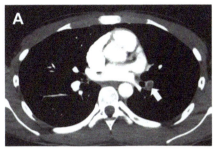 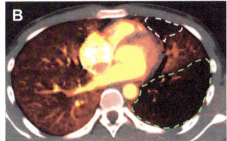

Fig. 10. (*A*) A 42 year old man with Factor V Leiden deficiency and acute chest pain. Axial CTPA shows an acute PE in the left lung, with most proximal involvement of the left lower lobe pulmonary artery (*arrow*). (*B*) A 42 year old man with Factor V Leiden deficiency and acute chest pain perfused blood volume PBV colored overlay on anatomic image of the same patient, at a slice inferior to (*A*), represents the iodine density. Note the perfusion defect in the left lower lobe (*dashed green line*). Also, note a separate perfusion defect in the lingula circumscribed (*dashed white line*), which is likely the result of a smaller thrombus below the resolution of CTPA.

angiography has demonstrated the highest diagnostic performance for PE in animal models.[39] Additionally, MECT offers prognostic value in patients with PE by identifying those at higher risk for major adverse events. The volume fraction of hypoperfused lung measured by MECT PBV was found to have good correlation with markers of right heart strain and moderate correlation with the Mastora score and right-to-left ventricle diameter ratio in a 4 chamber view.[40]

Another method for obtaining perfusion maps of the lungs on CTPA is subtraction CT. This technique involves acquiring both a precontrast image and a contrast-enhanced angiographic phase. A key advantage of this approach is that it does not necessitate hardware upgrades; however, it does rely on advanced motion correction software to align the unenhanced image with the enhanced CT image.[41,42] Incorporation of subtraction perfusion images into routine CTPA offers improvements over standard CTPA images and has shown comparable results to MECT iodine maps.[43]

PCCT represents the newest breakthrough in CT technology, offering potential enhancements for CTPA. PCCT uses energy-resolving detectors that count individual x-ray photons and measure their energy. This technology differs from conventional energy-integrating detectors (EIDs) by directly converting x-ray photons into electrical signals without the intermediate step of converting photons to visible light. The result is a higher CNR, improved spatial resolution, and optimized MECT imaging (**Fig. 11**A–C). PCCT reduces radiation exposure, corrects beam-hardening artifacts, and enhances the use of contrast agents, offering substantial improvements in diagnostic accuracy and quantitative imaging capabilities.[41] These advancements facilitate more precise imaging and material differentiation, positioning PCCT as a significant improvement over traditional CTPA methods. A study comparing PCCT and EID-CT for diagnosing acute PE found that PCCT provided MECT imaging for all patients, reduced acquisition time enabled by high helical pitch, and significantly lowered radiation dose by almost 50%. Additionally, PCCT resulted in fewer artifacts while providing perfusion maps in all patients.[44]

ARTIFICIAL INTELLIGENCE IN ACUTE PULMONARY EMBOLISM

Ever growing volumes of imaging studies due to easy availability of scanners, overuse of CT, and a global shortage of radiologists have resulted in delay in reporting urgent results for CTPA examinations and incidental acute PE on chest and abdominal CT scans performed for other reasons.[40,45,46] AI tools can support radiologists in the detection of PE as a second reader and by improving productivity and efficiency by accelerating workflows for the evaluation of PE.[47–49] The role of AI can be categorized into detection of PE, impact on clinical workflow, and prognostication.

ARTIFICIAL INTELLIGENCE IN DETECTION OF SUSPECTED ACUTE PULMONARY EMBOLISM

A number of retrospective studies using computer-aided detection (CAD) or AI algorithms have been described for detection of overlooked acute PE.[50–52] In a retrospective study, which involved review of CTPA scans by 3 radiologists, CAD identified 77% of PEs overlooked in clinical practice.[50] A study to evaluate the performance of Food and Drug Administration (FDA)-approved AI algorithm based on deep convolutional network for automatic detection of PE on CTPA examinations found a high diagnostic accuracy on a per

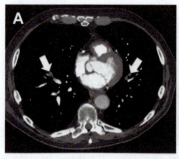 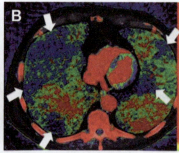 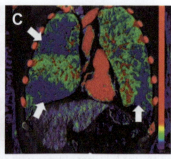

Fig. 11. (*A*) A 53 year old man with acute shortness of breath. Axial CTPA performed on a PCCT scanner shows multiple acute subsegmental acute PEs (*arrows*) in middle lobe and lingula. Note the clear delineation of the filling defects even in the lingula, a region commonly affected by cardiac pulsation. PCCT has inherently multi-energy capabilities. (*B*) A 53 year old man with acute shortness of breath axial overlayed iodine density maps shows multiple perfusion defects secondary to PE in the same patient (*arrows*). (*C*) A 53 year old man with acute shortness of breath coronal overlayed iodine density shows multiple perfusion defects secondary to PE in the same patient (*arrows*).

examination level and sensitivity and specificity of 92.7% and 95.5%, respectively[53] (**Fig. 12**A, B). The reference standard for per patient was based on the final written reports, and manual review of images for per finding. Another retrospective study showed that the same AI algorithms had higher sensitivity and specificity compared to the initial radiology report.[54]

The performance of the same commercial algorithm with those of emergency radiologists for diagnosing PE on CTPA in routine clinical practice showed significantly high sensitivity and negative predictive values (NPVs) with AI (92.6% vs 90% and 98.6% vs 98.1%, respectively).[55] AI missed 14 PEs detected by radiologists but flagged 19 PE cases overlooked by radiologists. In a subcohort with poor-to-average injection quality on CTPA, the AI algorithm showed improved diagnostic confidence of the radiologist.

Another study showed that this AI tool had high specificity for PE detection on CTPA examinations but lower sensitivity than in other studies, which could possibly be due to differences in patient populations, CT equipment, or acquisition protocols.[56]

In a prospective study, use of the earlier AI triage system to detect any PE on CTPA did not enhance radiologist accuracy or miss rate, and no difference was observed between radiologists and AI with respect to specificity and positive predictive value ($P=.78$ and $P=.91$, respectively). Although the sensitivity for the detection of subsegmental PE by the AI tool was lower, the miss rate was higher for radiologists without AI as compared with AI.[57] The same PE-AI triage model algorithm, however, showed similar performance on suboptimal CTPAs (marred by artifacts including motion artifacts or poor contrast opacification) and optimal CTPA examinations, a finding that supports a clinically

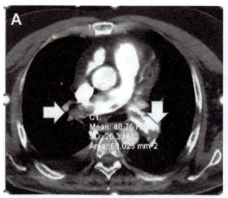 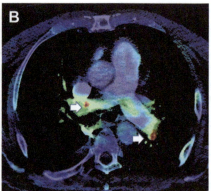

Fig. 12. (*A*) A 54 year old man with gastric cancer, and acute chest pain. Axial CTPA shows multiple central occlusive and nonocclusive emboli in the main pulmonary arteries and left inferior pulmonary trunk consistent. (*B*) Activation map shows the location determined by the AI algorithm corresponding to the acute PE at the same level.

meaningful sensitivity and high specificity regardless of diagnostic quality.[58]

ARTIFICIAL INTELLIGENCE IN DETECTION OF INCIDENTAL PULMONARY EMBOLISM

PE detected on imaging examinations performed for reasons other than suspected PE is referred to as incidental PE (IPE). The incidence of IPE ranges from 0.4% to 4.0% based on the patient population and type of CT scanner and has a high frequency in oncology patients up to 3.4%.[59] The risk of recurrent venous thromboembolism is also high in this group of patients, and IPE correlates with worse cancer prognosis and mortality.[60,61] Therefore, accurate detection of IPE is critical for timely management, as the presence of even isolated single or multiple subsegmental PEs may warrant treatment,[17] although treatment of such emboli remains debatable.

AI algorithms for detection of IPE on conventional contrast-enhanced chest CT (CECT) scans face a challenging task given the low frequency and large dataset validation requirement. Additionally CECT examinations are performed using different contrast medium bolus timing. Complex parenchymal disease and a wide range of additional findings such as enlarged lymph nodes, metastases, lung disease, or surgical changes may not have been present in the algorithm training dataset.

The performance of one AI algorithm was compared to the radiology reports in one study, and AI showed comparable performance with the radiologists with a high NPV (99.8% vs 99.9%, respectively).[47] AI flagged 4 IPE not mentioned in radiology reports and missed 7 IPE mentioned in clinical reports. The AI tool falsely flagged the examinations for acute PE in the setting of streak artifacts (Fig. 13A, B), lymphadenopathy (Fig. 14A, B), small nodules, pulmonary venous filling defect, and flow artifacts. AI missed emboli in complex parenchymal diseases, surgically altered anatomy, and in small caliber subsegmental vessels.

The performance of the same AI algorithm had a high sensitivity specificity of 91.6%, 99.7% respectively, and a 99.9% NPV in another study.[62] More than 80% of PE missed by AI was in the peripheral (segmental or subsegmental) vessels. Performance of the AI algorithms on abdominal CT scans that include the lung bases obtained during portal venous phase of contrast enhancement showed higher sensitivity for IPE compared to the original radiology report suggesting the AI algorithms can support radiologists by flagging the IPE in an otherwise routine busy daily workflow.[51]

IMPACT ON CLINICAL WORKFLOW

Rapid growth in imaging volumes and radiologist staff shortages have the potential to cause delay in interpretation of examinations with urgent findings, such as pulmonary emboli.[49] An AI algorithm, which identifies suspected PE and IPE with a high PPV and reprioritizes flagged studies to the top of the worklist, could have a significant impact on the workflow and result in timelier reporting of PE. Active reprioritization of the worklist with AI flagged positive has a superior impact on turnaround time of the reports as compared to widget interface when measuring turnaround time of the reports.[63] A widget is a notification chat box that pops with a list of positive examinations flagged by the AI tool in a past specific time interval and appears on the radiologists' ancillary monitor. The interface also includes the key images uploaded into the picture archiving and communication system.

A retrospective study found that reprioritization of the radiology worklist using an AI tool to flag suspected acute PE on CTPA resulted in reduced report turnaround by a mean of 12 minutes.[56] Another study looking at the performance of an AI algorithm for IPE detection in oncology patients showed that AI-assisted workflow prioritization reduced the median detection and notification time of IPE to just over 2 hours with a backlog of examinations of average 3 to 4 days.[62] In a prospective study, the mean wait time (time interval between the examination complete time by the technologist and the time point of the initiation of the report) decreased for PE-positive CTPA examinations (11.3 minutes with AI vs 16.7 minutes without AI).[57]

IMPACT ON PROGNOSIS

AI may contribute to risk stratification of patients with acute PE. Deep learning methods that accurately segment PE on CT and determine the clot burden have good correlation with the Qanadli scores and Mastora scores (rho 0.82 and 0.87, respectively), as well as with RV functional parameters on CTPA.[64–67] In a recent retrospective study of 101 patients with acute PE confirmed on CTPA, automated calculation of the RV/LV diameter ratio using AI post-processing software had good correlation correlated with manual analysis of RV/LV ratio (intraclass coefficient 0.78–0.83) and was attainable 87% of patients.[68]

BARRIERS TO ARTIFICIAL INTELLIGENCE INTEGRATION

Development, integration, and implementation of AI come with challenges. Large and heterogeneous

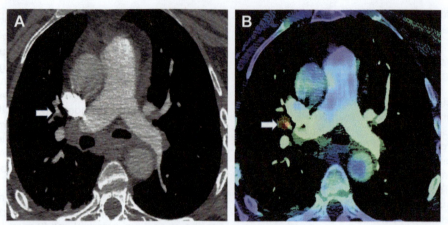

Fig. 13. (*A*) A 51 year old man with chest pain. Axial CTPA shows streak artifact from the dense contrast in the SVC creating an artifact simulating emboli in the right upper lobe anterior segmental branch. (*B*) A 51 year old man with chest pain. The AI algorithm flagged the examination falsely as positive for acute PE.

medical imaging datasets are important to limit inherent biases from age, sex, or technological factors. Inter-reader variability may affect accurate labeling of the pathology of interest in large anonymized high-quality annotated datasets for training with deep learning algorithms. It is imperative to have robust training, testing, and validation for the deep learning applications, notwithstanding the aspects of data privacy, ethical and regulatory issues.[69–71] Appropriate and recurrent monitoring of AI tools is mandatory following successful implementation in clinical practice given the impact on metric performance by patient population, prevalence of disease, comparable performance between the AI and radiologists, as well as automation bias.[72] Cost is an important challenge when considering AI clinical tools for licenses and reimbursement (not yet for the PE AI algorithm). Strong information technology infrastructure is important for seamless integration of AI. False-positive examinations can cause alert fatigue in radiologists, and AI optimization is important to limit that number.[73]

ARTIFICIAL INTELLIGENCE IN VENTILATION-PERFUSION SCINTIGRAPHY

Ventilation-perfusion (V/Q) scintigraphy is a noninvasive radiologic examination used to diagnose PE. The use of V/Q scintigraphy has substantially decreased due to a high percentage of indeterminate findings and increased use of CTPA.[74,75] Several qualitative assessment algorithms have been proposed and are used to interpret V/Q scans. The gestalt method is characterized as the most accurate, although this method is highly dependent on reader experience.[76] Many interpretation schemes have been proposed including the

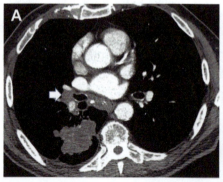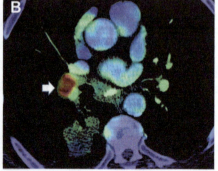

Fig. 14. (*A*) A 62 year old man with colon cancer, and metastasis to lung and lymph nodes. Axial CECT of the chest at the level of the right hilum shows enlarged right hilar (*arrow*) and sub-carinal lymphadenopathy, large mass in the right lower lobe, and small right pleural effusion. (*B*) A 62 year old man with colon cancer, and metastasis to lung and lymph nodes. False-positive acute PE flagged by AI. The activation map shows the location determined by the algorithm (*arrow*), which corresponds to an enlarged right hilar node.

Prospective Investigation of Pulmonary Embolism Diagnosis (PIOPED),[77] PIOPED II,[78] perfusion-only the Prospective Investigative Study of Acute Pulmonary Embolism Diagnosis (PISAPED),[79] and the European Association of Nuclear Medicine (EANM).[80]

The V/Q technique is composed of 2 components: the ventilation component (V) and the perfusion component (Q). Aerosols and inert gases can be used for ventilation imaging. Many institutions, guided by the Society of Nuclear Medicine and Molecular Imaging[81] and the American College of Radiology (ACR),[82] excluded the ventilation portion of the examination during the coronavirus disease 2019 (COVID-19) pandemic secondary to the concern of transmission of the disease through the ventilation systems. 99mTc-diethylene-triaminepentaacetic acid is the most commonly used aerosol and 133Xe is a noble gas available for ventilation scintigraphy. Xenon provides better physiologic evaluation of ventilation and is more sensitive for airway obstruction.[83] 99m Tc macro-aggregated albumin is the perfusion agent used in V/Q scan.[83,84] SPECT/CT is used to generate 3 dimensional data of pulmonary perfusion and can be correlated with CT for anatomic localization and anatomic findings of pulmonary disease such as pneumonia (Fig. 15A–D). Its usage is strongly recommended for perfusion imaging[80] by the EANM.

Visual assessment of a V/Q scan begins by tracking the lung periphery on perfusion images. Ventilation and radiologic examination are used for further characterization if abnormalities are identified on perfusion imaging. A perfusion abnormality, from a pulmonary embolus, causes a mismatched defect (perfusion defect without a ventilation defect). A triple match occurs when a matched V/Q defect corresponds with a radiographic abnormality, and although it is typically seen with pneumonia, infarction caused by acute PE can have a similar appearance. Triple matches in the lower lobe are more likely to be due to PE than triple matches in the upper lobes.[85] Localization of defects as segmental versus nonsegmental and size of defect play important role in interpretation and are included in the algorithmic interpretation criteria such as the Modified PIOPED II Criteria.[86]

V/Q scans were one of the earliest imaging examinations used for AI modeling, and specific AI models (validated by invasive pulmonary angiography) were reported to perform better than experienced radiologists for diagnosis of PE.[87,88] A recent systematic review reported 21 studies evaluating PE using shallow artificial neural networks. Ground truth labeling was determined by invasive pulmonary angiography and physician interpretation.[89]

Convolutional Neural Networks (CNNs) — a subset of AI used primarily for image recognition and processing — have a promising role in the diagnosis of PE and a potential to outperform the hard-coded or manual feature extraction for the ventilation and perfusion images. This is exemplified by an AI model that uses CNN-based texture features extracted from perfusion SPECT/CT images to detect PE with results of area under curve (AUCs) ranging from 0.86 to 0.98.[90] Future opportunities for AI in V/Q scintigraphy include image quality enhancement through artifact and noise removal, motion correction, and dose reduction.

MR ANGIOGRAPHY IN ACUTE PULMONARY EMBOLISM

MR angiography (MRA) is increasingly recognized as an alternative imaging modality for evaluation of acute PE, albeit in special situations. The lack of ionizing radiation and ability to obtain diagnostic images without administration of iodinated contrast agents portends a safer alternative diagnostic modality for patients with renal insufficiency or reactions to iodinated contrast.[91,92]

MRA has a high NPV in the detection of PE.[93] The technical success of MRA can vary significantly between institutions, based on experience and equipment quality. In experienced centers, the NPV of MRA for diagnosing PE may be as high as 97% at 3 months follow-up[94] to the effect that the modality may be utilized in routine use to diagnose PE (Fig. 16A, B). However, challenges like inadequate patient preparation, need for breath holding, or suboptimal contrast timing can compromise image quality[93], and longer acquisition times can limit its use in emergency settings.

The use of blood pool contrast agents, such as ferumoxytol (not currently labeled by the FDA), based on ultrasmall superparamagnetic iron oxide particles shows promising results in enhancing the performance of high-quality MRA for detecting PE. A recent multicenter registry has demonstrated that several ferumoxytol injections were well tolerated with no serious adverse reactions reported.[95] Furthermore, Starekova and colleagues[95] reported their experiences with ferumoxytol-enhanced MRA in 94 pregnant women demonstrating high quality and confidence scores for the diagnosis.

While CTPA remains the standard of care for the rapid diagnosis of PE due to its high sensitivity, specificity, and wide availability, MRA provides a valuable alternative in cases where CTPA is contraindicated.[93]

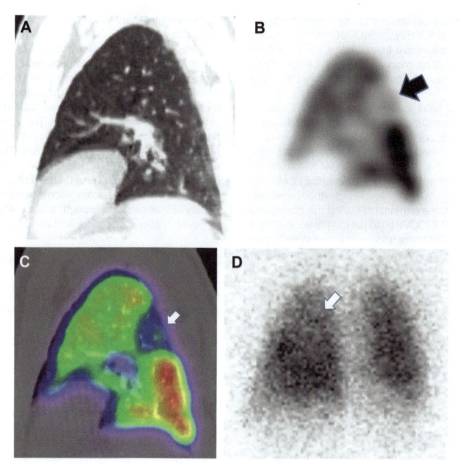

Fig. 15. (A) Sagittal reformatted CT image (lung window settings) shows no pulmonary opacity in a 34 year old man with lung transplant evaluation with SPECT-CT after 5.5 mCi of technietium-99m-MAA. (B) Sagittal SPECT shows perfusion defect in the superior segment of the left lower lobe (arrow). (C) Fused CT and SPECT images show perfusion defect in the superior segment of the left lower lobe. (D) Planar scintigraphy in left posterior oblique projection shows segmental perfusion defect in the superior segment of the left lower lobe (arrow).

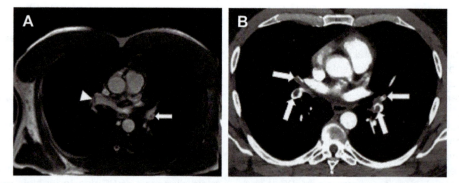

Fig. 16. (A) Diagnosis of PE on MRA. Unenhanced steady-state free precession imaging showing a hypointense filling defect in the basilar trunk of the left lower lobe pulmonary artery (arrow) and questionable filling defect at the bifurcation of the bronchus intermedius (arrowhead), suggestive of PE. (B) CTPA performed on the same day confirms multiple bilateral filling defects in segmental branches of the pulmonary arteries (arrows).

SUMMARY

Imaging plays a crucial role in the diagnosis and management of acute PE. Recent advances in CTPA techniques like MECT and PCCT offer faster scans with lower radiation dose while maintaining image quality. Various CT artifacts can mimic acute pulmonary emboli due to heterogeneous vascular opacification and rapid acquisition times, in the current state-of-the-art scanners. Radiologists should be able to recognize and manage these artifacts especially in critically sick patients. Recent times have also witnessed AI algorithms for detecting suspected or IPE with high diagnostic performance. In an era of exponential increase in the demand for imaging and a global shortage of radiologists, AI has the potential to act as a complementary tool to radiologists for improving patient care, and as a triage tool for worklist prioritization. However, integration of AI must positively affect clinical outcome and provide sufficient clinical improvement to justify its cost and timing. MRA is an alternative modality to CTPA in scenarios where radiation exposure is to be avoided or if patient is allergic to iodinated contrast.

REFERENCES

1. Jiménez D, Aujesky D, Díaz G, et al. Prognostic significance of deep vein thrombosis in patients presenting with acute symptomatic pulmonary embolism. Am J Respir Crit Care Med 2010;181(9): 983–91.
2. Konstantinides SV. Trends in incidence versus case fatality rates of pulmonary embolism: good news or bad news? Thromb Haemostasis 2016;115(2):233–5.
3. Kahn SR, de Wit K. Pulmonary embolism. N Engl J Med 2022;387(1):45–57.
4. Lehnert P, Lange T, Moller CH, et al. Acute pulmonary embolism in a national Danish cohort: increasing incidence and decreasing mortality. Thromb Haemostasis 2018;118(3):539–46.
5. Pagkalidou E, Doundoulakis I, Apostolidou-Kiouti F, et al. An overview of systematic reviews on imaging tests for diagnosis of pulmonary embolism applying different network meta-analytic methods. Hellenic J Cardiol 2024;76:88–98.
6. Krutman M, Wolosker N, Kuzniec S, et al. Risk of asymptomatic pulmonary embolism in patients with deep venous thrombosis. J Vasc Surg Venous Lymphat Disord 2013;1(4):370–5.
7. Schrecengost JE, LeGallo RD, Boyd JC, et al. Comparison of diagnostic accuracies in outpatients and hospitalized patients of D-dimer testing for the evaluation of suspected pulmonary embolism. Clin Chem 2003;49(9):1483–90.
8. Worsley DF, Alavi A, Aronchick JM, et al. Chest radiographic findings in patients with acute pulmonary embolism: observations from the PIOPED Study. Radiology 1993;189(1):133–6.
9. Remy-Jardin M, Remy J, Wattinne L, et al. Central pulmonary thromboembolism: diagnosis with spiral volumetric CT with the single-breath-hold technique–comparison with pulmonary angiography. Radiology 1992;185(2):381–7.
10. Stein PD, Fowler SE, Goodman LR, et al. Multidetector computed tomography for acute pulmonary embolism. N Engl J Med 2006;354(22):2317–27.
11. Patel P, Patel P, Bhatt M, et al. Systematic review and meta-analysis of test accuracy for the diagnosis of suspected pulmonary embolism. Blood Adv 2020; 4(18):4296–311.
12. Nguyen ET, Hague C, Manos D, et al. Canadian society of thoracic radiology/Canadian association of radiologists best practice guidance for investigation of acute pulmonary embolism, Part 1: acquisition and safety considerations. Can Assoc Radiol J 2022;73(1):203–13.
13. Schönfeld T, Seitz P, Krieghoff C, et al. High-pitch CT pulmonary angiography (CTPA) with ultra-low contrast medium volume for the detection of pulmonary embolism: a comparison with standard CTPA. Eur Radiol 2024;34(3):1921–31.
14. Hou DJ, Tso DK, Davison C, et al. Clinical utility of ultra-high pitch dual source thoracic CT imaging of acute pulmonary embolism in the emergency department: are we one step closer towards a non-gated triple rule out? Eur J Radiol 2013;82(10): 1793–8.
15. Wittram C. How I do it: CT pulmonary angiography. AJR Am J Roentgenol 2007;188(5):1255–61.
16. Newnham M, Turner AM. Diagnosis and treatment of subsegmental pulmonary embolism. World J Respirol 2019;9(3):30–4.
17. Le Gal G, Kovacs MJ, Bertoletti L, et al. Risk for recurrent venous thromboembolism in patients with subsegmental pulmonary embolism managed without anticoagulation : a multicenter prospective cohort study. Ann Intern Med 2022;175(1):29–35.
18. Furlan A, Aghayev A, Chang CC, et al. Short-term mortality in acute pulmonary embolism: clot burden and signs of right heart dysfunction at CT pulmonary angiography. Radiology 2012;265(1):283–93. https://doi.org/10.1148/radiol.12110802.
19. Mastora I, Remy-Jardin M, Masson P, et al. Severity of acute pulmonary embolism: evaluation of a new spiral CT angiographic score in correlation with echocardiographic data. Eur Radiol 2003;13(1):29–35.
20. Chornenki NLJ, Poorzargar K, Shanjer M, et al. Detection of right ventricular dysfunction in acute pulmonary embolism by computed tomography or echocardiography: a systematic review and meta-analysis. J Thromb Haemostasis 2021;19(10):2504–13.

21. Chaosuwannakit N, Soontrapa W, Makarawate P, et al. Importance of computed tomography pulmonary angiography for predict 30-day mortality in acute pulmonary embolism patients. Eur J Radiol Open 2021;8:100340.
22. Apfaltrer P, Walter T, Gruettner J, et al. Prediction of adverse clinical outcome in patients with acute pulmonary embolism: evaluation of high-sensitivity troponin I and quantitative CT parameters. Eur J Radiol 2013;82(3):563–7.
23. Beyls C, Vial J, Lefebvre T, et al. Prognostic value of right ventricular dilatation on computed tomography pulmonary angiogram for predicting adverse clinical events in severe COVID-19 pneumonia. Front Med (Lausanne) 2023;10:1213775.
24. Yang F, Chen R, Yang Y, et al. Predictive value of pulmonary artery distensibility for short-term adverse clinical outcomes in patients with acute pulmonary embolism. Clin Appl Thromb Hemost 2024;30. 10760296231224344.
25. Lyhne MD, Schultz JG, MacMahon PJ, et al. Septal bowing and pulmonary artery diameter on computed tomography pulmonary angiography are associated with short-term outcomes in patients with acute pulmonary embolism. Emerg Radiol 2019;26(6):623–30.
26. Kallianos KG, Hope MD, Henry TS. Approach to abnormal chest computed tomography contrast enhancement in the hospitalized patient. Radiol Clin North Am 2020;58(1):93–103.
27. Wittram C, Maher MM, Halpern EF, et al. Attenuation of acute and chronic pulmonary emboli. Radiology 2005;235(3):1050–4.
28. Henry TS, Hammer MM, Little BP, et al. Smoke: how to differentiate flow-related artifacts from pathology on thoracic computed tomographic angiography. J Thorac Imaging 2019;34(5):W109–20.
29. Main C, Abbas A, Shambrook JS, et al. Clot or not? An unusual case of false positive CTPA and an approach to diagnosis. BJR Case Rep 2016;3(1): 20160021.
30. Damm R, Mohnike K, Gazis A, et al. Improvement of contrast media enhancement in CTA evaluating pulmonary embolism by utilizing 'delayed' bolus tracking in the descending aorta. Pol J Radiol 2016;81:422–7.
31. Rajiah P, Parakh A, Kay F, et al. Update on multienergy CT: physics, principles, and applications. Radiographics 2020;40(5):1284–308.
32. Grant KL, Flohr TG, Krauss B, et al. Assessment of an advanced image-based technique to calculate virtual monoenergetic computed tomographic images from a dual-energy examination to improve contrast-to-noise ratio in examinations using iodinated contrast media. Invest Radiol 2014;49(9): 586–92.
33. Wannasopha Y, Leesmidt K, Srisuwan T, et al. Value of low-keV virtual monoenergetic plus dual-energy computed tomographic imaging for detection of acute pulmonary embolism. PLoS One 2022; 17(11):e0277060.
34. Thieme SF, Hoegl S, Nikolaou K, et al. Pulmonary ventilation and perfusion imaging with dual-energy CT. Eur Radiol 2010;20(12):2882–9.
35. Fuld MK, Halaweish AF, Haynes SE, et al. Pulmonary perfused blood volume with dual-energy CT as surrogate for pulmonary perfusion assessed with dynamic multidetector CT. Radiology 2013;267(3):747–56.
36. Meinel FG, Graef A, Sommer WH, et al. Influence of vascular enhancement, age and gender on pulmonary perfused blood volume quantified by dual-energy-CTPA. Eur J Radiol 2013;82(9):1565–70.
37. Thieme SF, Becker CR, Hacker M, et al. Dual energy CT for the assessment of lung perfusion–correlation to scintigraphy. Eur J Radiol 2008;68(3):369–74.
38. Thieme SF, Graute V, Nikolaou K, et al. Dual Energy CT lung perfusion imaging–correlation with SPECT/CT. Eur J Radiol 2012;81(2):360–5.
39. Zhang LJ, Chai X, Wu SY, et al. Detection of pulmonary embolism by dual energy CT: correlation with perfusion scintigraphy and histopathological findings in rabbits. Eur Radiol 2009;19(12):2844–54.
40. Apfaltrer P, Bachmann V, Meyer M, et al. Prognostic value of perfusion defect volume at dual energy CTA in patients with pulmonary embolism: correlation with CTA obstruction scores, CT parameters of right ventricular dysfunction and adverse clinical outcome. Eur J Radiol 2012;81(11):3592–7.
41. Grob D, Oostveen LJ, Prokop M, et al. Imaging of pulmonary perfusion using subtraction CT angiography is feasible in clinical practice. Eur Radiol 2019;29(3):1408–14.
42. Grob D, Smit E, Prince J, et al. Iodine maps from subtraction CT or dual-energy CT to detect pulmonary emboli with CT angiography: a multiple-observer study. Radiology 2019;292(1):197–205.
43. Willemink MJ, Persson M, Pourmorteza A, et al. Photon-counting CT: technical principles and clinical prospects. Radiology 2018;289(2):293–312.
44. Remy-Jardin M, Oufriche I, Guiffault L, et al. Diagnosis of acute pulmonary embolism: when photon-counting-detector CT replaces energy-integrating-detector CT in daily routine. Eur Radiol 2024. https://doi.org/10.1007/s00330-024-10724-5.
45. Lim KY, Kligerman SJ, Lin CT, et al. Missed pulmonary embolism on abdominal CT. AJR Am J Roentgenol 2014;202(4):738–43.
46. Jha S. Value of triage by artificial intelligence. Acad Radiol 2020;27(1):153–5.
47. Batra K, Xi Y, Al-Hreish KM, et al. Detection of incidental pulmonary embolism on conventional contrast-enhanced chest CT: comparison of an artificial intelligence algorithm and clinical reports. AJR Am J Roentgenol 2022;219(6):895–902.
48. Kapoor N, Lacson R, Khorasani R. Workflow applications of artificial intelligence in radiology and an

overview of available tools. J Am Coll Radiol 2020; 17(11):1363–70.
49. Omofoye TS, Vlahos I, Marom EM, et al. Backlogs in formal interpretation of radiology examinations: a pilot global survey. Clin Imaging 2024;106:110049.
50. Kligerman SJ, Lahiji K, Galvin JR, et al. Missed pulmonary emboli on CT angiography: assessment with pulmonary embolism-computer-aided detection. AJR Am J Roentgenol 2014;202(1):65–73.
51. Langius-Wiffen E, de Jong PA, Mohamed Hoesein FA, et al. Added value of an artificial intelligence algorithm in reducing the number of missed incidental acute pulmonary embolism in routine portal venous phase chest CT. Eur Radiol 2024;34(1):367–73.
52. Wildman-Tobriner B, Ngo L, Mammarappallil JG, et al. Missed incidental pulmonary embolism: harnessing artificial intelligence to assess prevalence and improve quality improvement opportunities. J Am Coll Radiol 2021;18(7):992–9.
53. Weikert T, Winkel DJ, Bremerich J, et al. Automated detection of pulmonary embolism in CT pulmonary angiograms using an AI-powered algorithm. Eur Radiol 2020;30(12):6545–53.
54. Langius-Wiffen E, de Jong PA, Hoesein FAM, et al. Retrospective batch analysis to evaluate the diagnostic accuracy of a clinically deployed AI algorithm for the detection of acute pulmonary embolism on CTPA. Insights Imaging 2023;14(1):102.
55. Cheikh AB, Gorincour G, Nivet H, et al. How artificial intelligence improves radiological interpretation in suspected pulmonary embolism. Eur Radiol 2022;32(9):5831–42.
56. Batra K, Xi Y, Bhagwat S, et al. Radiologist worklist reprioritization using artificial intelligence: impact on report turnaround times for CTPA examinations positive for acute pulmonary embolism. AJR Am J Roentgenol 2023;221(3):324–33.
57. Rothenberg SA, Savage CH, Abou Elkassem A, et al. Prospective evaluation of AI triage of pulmonary emboli on CT pulmonary angiograms. Radiology 2023;309(1):e230702.
58. Ebrahimian S, Digumarthy SR, Homayounieh F, et al. Predictive values of AI-based triage model in suboptimal CT pulmonary angiography. Clin Imaging 2022;86:25–30.
59. Meyer HJ, Wienke A, Surov A. Incidental pulmonary embolism in oncologic patients-a systematic review and meta-analysis. Support Care Cancer 2021;29(3):1293–302.
60. Klok FA, Huisman MV. Management of incidental pulmonary embolism. Eur Respir J 2017;49(6):1700275.
61. Abdel-Razeq HN, Mansour AH, Ismael YM. Incidental pulmonary embolism in cancer patients: clinical characteristics and outcome—a comprehensive cancer center experience. Vasc Health Risk Manag 2011;7:153–8.
62. Topff L, Ranschaert ER, Bartels-Rutten A, et al. Artificial intelligence tool for detection and worklist prioritization reduces time to diagnosis of incidental pulmonary embolism at CT. Radiol Cardiothorac Imaging 2023;5(2):e220163.
63. O'Neill TJ, Xi Y, Stehel E, et al. Active reprioritization of the reading worklist using artificial intelligence has a beneficial effect on the turnaround time for interpretation of head CT with intracranial hemorrhage. Radiol Artif Intell 2020;3(2):e200024.
64. Liu Z, Yuan H, Wang H. CAM-Wnet: an effective solution for accurate pulmonary embolism segmentation. Med Phys 2022;49(8):5294–303.
65. Aydın N, Cihan Ç, Çelik Ö, et al. Segmentation of acute pulmonary embolism in computed tomography pulmonary angiography using the deep learning method. Tuberk Toraks 2023;71(2):131–7.
66. Liu W, Liu M, Guo X, et al. Evaluation of acute pulmonary embolism and clot burden on CTPA with deep learning. Eur Radiol 2020;30(6):3567–75.
67. Zhang H, Cheng Y, Chen Z, et al. Clot burden of acute pulmonary thromboembolism: comparison of two deep learning algorithms, Qanadli score, and Mastora score. Quant Imaging Med Surg 2022;12(1):66–79.
68. Foley RW, Glenn-Cox S, Rossdale J, et al. Automated calculation of the right ventricle to left ventricle ratio on CT for the risk stratification of patients with acute pulmonary embolism. Eur Radiol 2021;31(8):6013–20.
69. Lee SM, Seo JB, Yun J, et al. Deep learning applications in chest radiography and computed tomography: current state of the art. J Thorac Imaging 2019;34(2):75–85.
70. Rajpurkar P, Chen E, Banerjee O, et al. AI in health and medicine. Nat Med 2022;28(1):31–8.
71. European Society of Radiology (ESR). What the radiologist should know about artificial intelligence - an ESR white paper. Insights Imaging 2019;10(1):44.
72. Daye D, Wiggins WF, Lungren MP, et al. Implementation of clinical artificial intelligence in radiology: who decides and how? Radiology 2022;305(3):555–63.
73. Mendelson EB. Artificial intelligence in breast imaging: potentials and limitations. AJR Am J Roentgenol 2019;212(2):293–9.
74. Bonnefoy PB, Prevot N, Mehdipoor G, et al. Ventilation/perfusion (V/Q) scanning in contemporary patients with pulmonary embolism: utilization rates and predictors of use in a multinational study. J Thromb Thrombolysis 2022;53(4):829–40.
75. Wang RC, Miglioretti DL, Marlow EC, et al. Trends in imaging for suspected pulmonary embolism across US health care systems, 2004 to 2016. JAMA Netw Open 2020;3(11):e2026930.
76. Hagen PJ, Hartmann IJ, Hoekstra OS, et al. How to use a gestalt interpretation for ventilation-perfusion lung scintigraphy. J Nucl Med 2002;43(10):1317–23.

77. PIOPED Investigators. Value of the ventilation/perfusion scan in acute pulmonary embolism. Results of the prospective investigation of pulmonary embolism diagnosis (PIOPED). JAMA 1990;263(20): 2753–9.
78. Gottschalk A, Stein PD, Goodman LR, et al. Overview of prospective investigation of pulmonary embolism diagnosis II. Semin Nucl Med 2002;32(3): 173–82.
79. Miniati M, Pistolesi M, Marini C, et al. Value of perfusion lung scan in the diagnosis of pulmonary embolism: results of the prospective investigative study of acute pulmonary embolism diagnosis (PISA-PED). Am J Respir Crit Care Med 1996;154(5):1387–93.
80. Bajc M, Neilly JB, Miniati M, et al. EANM guidelines for ventilation/perfusion scintigraphy: Part 1. Pulmonary imaging with ventilation/perfusion single photon emission tomography. Eur J Nucl Med Mol Imaging 2009;36(8):1356–70.
81. SNMMI Statement. COVID-19 and ventilation/perfusion (V/Q) lung studies. J Nucl Med Technol 2021; 49(2):12A.
82. Davenport MS, Bruno MA, Iyer RS, et al. ACR statement on safe resumption of routine radiology care during the coronavirus disease 2019 (COVID-19) pandemic. J Am Coll Radiol 2020;17(7):839–44.
83. Parker JA, Coleman RE, Grady E, et al. SNM practice guideline for lung scintigraphy 4.0. J Nucl Med Technol 2012;40(1):57–65.
84. Worsley DF, Kim CK, Alavi A, et al. Detailed analysis of patients with matched ventilation-perfusion defects and chest radiographic opacities. J Nucl Med 1993;34(11):1851–3.
85. Sostman HD, Stein PD, Gottschalk A, et al. Acute pulmonary embolism: sensitivity and specificity of ventilation-perfusion scintigraphy in PIOPED II study. Radiology 2008;246(3):941–6.
86. Scott JA, Palmer EL, Fischman AJ. How well can radiologists using neural network software diagnose pulmonary embolism? AJR Am J Roentgenol 2000; 175(2):399–405.
87. Tourassi GD, Floyd CE, Coleman RE. Acute pulmonary embolism: cost-effectiveness analysis of the effect of artificial neural networks on patient care. Radiology 1998;206(1):81–8.
88. Jabbarpour A, Ghassel S, Lang J, et al. The past, present, and future role of artificial intelligence in ventilation/perfusion scintigraphy: a systematic review. Semin Nucl Med 2023;53(6):752–65.
89. Aloysius N,GM. A review on deep convolutional neural networks. In: IEEE international conference on communication and signal processing, ICCSP. 2017. p. 588–92.
90. Benson DG, Schiebler ML, Repplinger MD, et al. Contrast-enhanced pulmonary MRA for the primary diagnosis of pulmonary embolism: current state of the art and future directions. Br J Radiol 2017; 90(1074):20160901.
91. Dillman JR, Ellis JH, Cohan RH, et al. Frequency and severity of acute allergic-like reactions to gadolinium-containing i.v. contrast media in children and adults. AJR Am J Roentgenol 2007;189(6):1533–8.
92. Stein PD, Chenevert TL, Fowler SE, et al. Gadolinium-enhanced magnetic resonance angiography for pulmonary embolism: a multicenter prospective study (PIOPED III). Ann Intern Med 2010;152(7): 434–43. W142-3.
93. Schiebler ML, Nagle SK, François CJ, et al. Effectiveness of MR angiography for the primary diagnosis of acute pulmonary embolism: clinical outcomes at 3 months and 1 year. J Magn Reson Imag 2013;38(4): 914–25.
94. Nguyen KL, Yoshida T, Kathuria-Prakash N, et al. Multicenter safety and practice for off-label diagnostic use of ferumoxytol in MRI. Radiology 2019; 293(3):554–64.
95. Starekova J, Nagle SK, Schiebler ML, et al. Pulmonary MRA during pregnancy: early experience with ferumoxytol. J Magn Reson Imag 2023;57(6):1815–8.

Imaging of Chronic Thromboembolic Pulmonary Hypertension

Lewis D. Hahn, MD, Jonathan H. Chung, MD*

KEYWORDS

- CTEPH • Pulmonary embolism • Pulmonary hypertension • CT • Perfusion • Dual energy

KEY POINTS

- CT pulmonary angiography (CTPA) can be highly sensitive for detecting CTEPH, but the diagnosis is frequently missed by radiologists.
- Imaging findings of chronic thromboembolic pulmonary disease (CTEPD) differ from those of acute pulmonary embolism, though both chronic and acute disease may coexist on CTPA.
- Hypoperfusion can help pinpoint areas of CTEPD, a process that may be enhanced by spectral imaging techniques.
- Preoperative imaging aims to assess the extent of disease and identify other factors that could impact treatment decisions.
- Conditions that can mimic CTEPH include acute pulmonary embolism, in situ thrombus, pulmonary artery sarcoma, vasculitis, and fibrosing mediastinitis.

INTRODUCTION

Chronic thromboembolic pulmonary hypertension (CTEPH) is a form of pulmonary hypertension caused by prolonged obstruction of the pulmonary arteries by organized thromboemboli.[1] Each year, approximately 600,000 Americans experience an acute pulmonary embolism. While the majority of cases resolve, about 1% to 5% result in persistent thromboembolism and CTEPH.[2–4] Although a relatively rare disease, CTEPH is frequently missed both clinically and on imaging, particularly on CT pulmonary angiogram (CTPA). A recent position paper by the Fleischner Society highlighted the educational gap contributing to this underdiagnosis.[5] CTEPH is a treatable condition with surgical, endovascular, and medical interventions that can improve both survival and quality of life, making it crucial for radiologists to recognize the imaging findings of this disease.

This article will discuss imaging of CTEPH, with particular emphasis on CTPA. We will first discuss the clinical presentation and pathophysiology of CTEPH, followed by a review of normal pulmonary arterial anatomy and CTPA technique. Finally, we will describe the imaging features of CTEPH and its mimics.

CLINICAL PRESENTATION AND PATHOPHYSIOLOGY

The most common presenting symptoms of CTEPH are dyspnea on exertion and fatigue, which are nonspecific, likely contributing to underdiagnosis.[6,7] In the setting of right heart failure, patients may additionally experience related symptoms including lower extremity swelling, abdominal distension, chest pressure, and syncope, but these are less common presenting symptoms.[8] Similarly, hemoptysis related to

Department of Radiology, University of California San Diego, La Jolla, CA, USA
* Corresponding author.
E-mail address: jherochung@health.ucsd.edu

bronchial artery hypertrophy is a less-frequent presenting symptom.

Risk factors for CTEPH partially overlap with those for acute pulmonary embolism and include malignancy, chronic inflammatory states (eg, chronic infection from indwelling catheters), prior splenectomy, and hypothyroidism.[1] While antiphospholipid antibodies and lupus anticoagulant and coagulopathies related to elevated factor VIII, von Willebrand factor, and abnormal fibrinogen are associated with CTEPH, the most common inherited thrombotic risk factors such as protein C deficiency and protein S deficiency interestingly are not.[9]

Approximately 75% of patients with CTEPH have a history of acute pulmonary embolism, suggesting that most cases arise from the failure of acute emboli to resorb. While acute pulmonary embolism primarily consists of red blood cells, platelets, and fibrin, failure to resolve leads to infiltration by inflammatory cells, which organize the clot and deposit extracellular matrix proteins such as fibrin and elastin. This process results in a chronic thrombus that is inherently different in composition from acute pulmonary embolism.[10] In addition to obstructive thrombi, patients with CTEPH also develop a microvasculopathy, likely due to prolonged exposure to elevated pressures and associated shear stress.[6] In unobstructed pulmonary arteries, this is simply due to pulmonary hypertension, and in obstructed pulmonary arteries, it results from bronchial collateral vessels with systemic pressure.

CTEPH specifically refers to patients with chronic thromboembolism and pulmonary hypertension. Recent guidelines from the European Respiratory Society have proposed the term chronic thromboembolic pulmonary disease (CTEPD) to describe patients with chronic thromboembolism, with or without pulmonary hypertension at rest.[11] However, the term chronic thromboembolic disease (CTED) is still frequently used to describe patients with chronic thromboembolism without pulmonary hypertension.

NORMAL ANATOMY

Accurate knowledge of the pulmonary arterial tree is essential for identifying and characterizing thromboembolic disease. In patients with CTEPH, occluded or diminutive pulmonary arteries can easily be overlooked if not specifically included in the search pattern.

The main pulmonary artery (PA) bifurcates into the right and left pulmonary arteries. The right PA continues as the interlobar artery beyond the first branch to the right upper lobe PA, usually the truncus anterior. Variable terminology has been used to describe the segment of the left PA distal to the first left upper lobe PA, with some still describing it as the left PA, and others using the term left descending or interlobar PA.

Segmental pulmonary arteries are named according to the bronchopulmonary segments they supply and usually run parallel to the segmental bronchi. However, many anatomic variations exist.[12–14] For accurate identification of segmental pulmonary arteries, it can be useful to first locate a bronchopulmonary segment and then trace the course of its dominant pulmonary arterial supply.

The right upper lobe consists of 3 segments supplied by the apical (A1), posterior (A2), and anterior (A3) segmental arteries. The apical and anterior segmental arteries most often share a common trunk, called the truncus anterior, while the posterior segmental artery arises separately from the interlobar artery. The right middle lobe has 2 segments supplied by lateral (A4) and medial (A5) segmental branches, which may have a common trunk. The right lower lobe superior segmental artery (A6) typically originates at or proximal to the takeoff of the right middle lobe arteries.[12] After giving off these branches, the interlobar artery continues as the right lower lobe basal trunk, which supplies the medial basal (A7), anterior basal (A8), lateral basal (A9), and posterior basal (A10) segmental arteries. The medial and anterior basal arteries (A7 + A8) usually arise from one trunk, while the lateral and posterior basal arteries (A9 + A10) arise from another.

The left upper lobe consists of the apicoposterior (A1–A2) and anterior (A3) segments, which may arise from separate segmental arteries or a common trunk. The superior (A4) and inferior (A5) lingular arteries typically share a common trunk but may arise separately. Similar to the right side, the left lower lobe superior segmental artery (A6) may arise at or proximal to the takeoff of the lingular pulmonary arteries. Beyond the A6 takeoff, the basal segmental arteries vary in their branching patterns, but most commonly, there are 2 trunks: one supplying the anteromedial basal segments (A7–A8) and the other supplying the lateral basal (A9) and posterior basal (A10) segments.

CT IMAGING TECHNIQUE

CTPA technique for CTEPH is similar to that used for acute pulmonary embolism. Typically, 75 to 100 mL of iodinated contrast is injected at 4 to 6 mL/s with adjustments based on patient body mass index.[15–18] A test bolus or automated bolus triggering is used to determine the scan delay with the region of interest usually placed in the main PA. In cases of slow flow due to pulmonary hypertension or left-sided heart failure, placing the region of interest in the left atrium may help ensure better opacification of the distal pulmonary arteries. Electrocardiogram (ECG)-gating is generally not required. Scanning is performed in a caudocranial direction, as the lower lobes are more prone to motion artifacts due to greater respiratory excursion compared to the upper lobes. This approach also reduces streak artifacts caused by contrast inflow into the superior vena cava (SVC).[17,19]

A key aspect of CTPA for CTEPH is using the thinnest possible slice thickness, typically 0.625 to 1.0 mm, to avoid the partial volume averaging that can obscure linear chronic thromboemboli. At our institution, we also reconstruct 3 plane maximum intensity projection (MIP) images at a thickness of 7 to 10 mm, which are useful for identifying small or occluded vessels.

When available, spectral imaging techniques, that is, dual-energy CT or photon counting CT, should be used for the identification of perfusion defects. At our institution, source iodine map images are used to generate 3 plane colorized postprocessed iodine maps reconstructed at a thickness of 12 mm. Although most institutions perform a single-phase CT, some have suggested the use of dual-phase CT for patients with known CTEPH to better evaluate collateral vessels, which can help differentiate acute from chronic disease.[20] Additionally, this technique may help distinguish between artifacts such as contrast "smoke" and true thromboembolic disease.

IMAGING FINDINGS/PATHOLOGY
V/Q Scan

V/Q is currently the screening modality of choice to exclude CTEPD.[11] While V/Q scan is reported to have a sensitivity of 96% to 97% and specificity of 90% to 95%,[13,14] V/Q scan may underestimate the extent of disease in cases of nonocclusive thromboembolism.[15] When available, single photon emission computed tomography - computed tomography (SPECT-CT) is preferred over planar imaging, as planar imaging has limitations such as overlapping pulmonary segments, adjacent lung shine-through, and challenges in assessing the size of defects.[5,16–18]

The interpretation of V/Q scans for CTEPD follows a similar approach to V/Q scans for acute pulmonary embolism, using the modified prospective investigation of pulmonary embolism diagnosis II (PIOPED II) criteria. While small mismatched perfusion defects do not exclude CTEPH, most CTEPH cases display moderate (25%–75% of a bronchopulmonary segment) or large (>75%) mismatched perfusion defects (Fig. 1). When mismatches in both ventilation and perfusion are detected, further

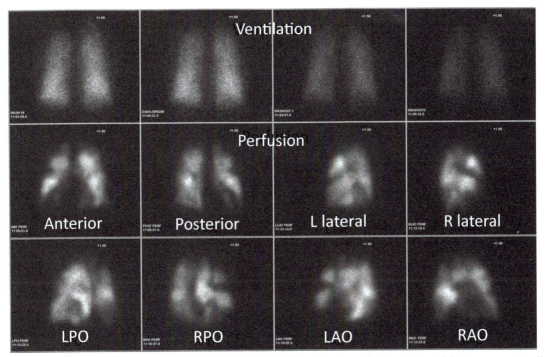

Fig. 1. V/Q scan of a 59 year old man with CTEPH. Large, bilateral mismatched perfusion defects are seen in all lobes, greater in the lower lobes.

evaluation with anatomic imaging is essential to assess the full extent of the disease, evaluate lung parenchyma abnormalities, or identify potential CTEPH mimics. Several other conditions can cause vascular obstruction with preserved airflow, further discussed in the CTEPH mimics section.

CT Pulmonary Angiogram

The pulmonary arterial filling defects of CTEPD on CTPA can often be distinguished from acute pulmonary embolism based on their morphology. Linear filling defects called "bands" are indicative of chronic rather than acute pulmonary embolism. Multiple bands joining together are called "webs" (Fig. 2A). Chronic thromboemboli are usually eccentrically positioned within the vessel, abutting the vessel wall, in contrast to the more centrally located acute emboli[15] (Fig. 2B, C). The margins of chronic emboli are usually concave, whereas acute emboli tend to have convex margins (Fig. 3A, B). Consequently, chronic thromboemboli form an obtuse angle with the vessel wall, while acute emboli form an acute angle.

In all cases of CTEPH, occluded vessels with decreased caliber are observed (Fig. 2C, D). In some cases, such vessels may be so diminutive that they appear to be "absent"; in this situation, it can be helpful to use lung windows and trace the bronchi to infer the presence of occluded vessels. In contrast, pulmonary arteries affected by occlusive acute pulmonary embolism will have a normal or increased caliber (Fig. 3C). CT imaging can underestimate thromboembolic disease because organized thrombus may be contracted and strongly adherent to the vessel wall, making it difficult to visualize (Fig. 4A, B). In fact, some cases of CTEPH will demonstrate no obvious pulmonary arterial filling defects, and it is solely the observation of reduced vessel caliber and distal occlusions, which suggests the diagnosis. This is particularly true in patients with prior splenectomy, who often only have isolated segmental and subsegmental disease (Fig. 5A–C). The presence of splenectomy in a patient being evaluated for CTEPH should prompt scrutiny of subsegmental vessel caliber, even if no obvious defects are visible on initial review.

The presence of acute pulmonary embolism does not rule out concurrent chronic disease. Many patients with CTEPH have repeated acute pulmonary embolism events, and CT can reveal findings of acute, subacute, and CTED simultaneously (Fig. 6). Retrospective review of CTPA at the time of initial acute pulmonary embolism diagnosis in patients with CTEPH often shows evidence of chronic thromboembolism, which is a common reason for missed diagnoses.[3]

Compensatory bronchial artery hypertrophy is often seen in patients with CTEPH. These arteries most often arise from the aorta but can also arise from the great vessels, intercostal arteries, and occasionally the coronary arteries. Large bronchial arteries can lead to retrograde perfusion of the

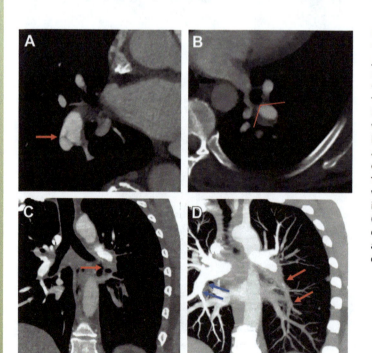

Fig. 2. Findings of CTEPD. (A) Axial CTPA image with multiple linear bands joining together to form a web in the right lower lobe basal trunk. (B) Axial CTPA image demonstrating eccentric thrombus with concave margin forming an obtuse angle with the vessel wall in the common trunk of the left lower lobe lateral and basal segmental arteries. (C) Coronal CTPA image demonstrating occlusive thrombus in the left descending pulmonary artery with concave margin. (D) Corresponding maximum intensity projection (MIP) image demonstrates diminutive caliber of the downstream pulmonary arteries (red arrows) relative to the contralateral side (blue arrows).

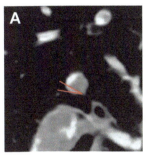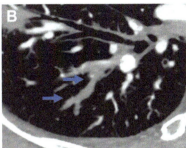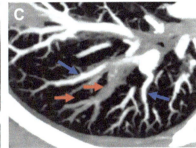

Fig. 3. Acute pulmonary embolism. (A) Acute pulmonary embolism has a convex margin, which forms an acute angle relative to the vessel wall. (B) In acute pulmonary embolism, the pulmonary artery is normal or increased in size. (C) Axial MIP image demonstrating enlarged caliber of the occluded pulmonary artery (red arrows) relative to adjacent patent subsegmental vessels (blue arrows).

pulmonary arteries, resulting in "smoke artifact" from unopacified blood if contrast does not sufficiently opacify the systemic arteries. The identification of large bronchial arteries is important because retrograde blood flow into the pulmonary arteries during cardiopulmonary bypass can obscure the surgical field during pulmonary thromboendarterectomy (PTE) surgery.[21]

Evaluation of the lung parenchyma can be useful to identify chronic thromboembolism. Mosaic perfusion is often pronounced in cases of CTEPH, and areas of hypoperfused lung can help direct attention to chronic thromboemboli in the corresponding pulmonary arteries (Fig. 7A, B). Even without dedicated iodine maps, mosaic perfusion can still be observed on single-energy CT images. Areas of normal or hyperperfusion may also be seen in regions without thromboembolic disease due to blood flow redistribution. Mosaic perfusion in CTEPD needs to be distinguished from mosaic perfusion due to small airways disease and hypoxic vasoconstriction. In such cases, the presence of large airways disease, as suggested by bronchial wall thickening or mucus plugging, along with the absence of thromboemboli, suggests airways disease as the cause of mosaic perfusion. However, bronchiectasis can occur with both CTEPH and airways disease, and its presence alone is not useful for differentiation. Mosaic perfusion is common in CTEPH, but in patients with CTEPD without pulmonary hypertension, it may be less conspicuous, particularly in nonobstructive cases. Finally, infarcts or peripheral scarring representing sequelae of infarcts are frequently observed in patients with CTEPH and an unexpected finding in patients with small airways disease.

Although right heart catheterization is required for a definitive CTEPH diagnosis, most patients with CTEPH will demonstrate CT evidence of pulmonary hypertension (Fig. 8A, B). According to the Fleischner Society, a PA diameter greater than 32 mm or a PA-to-aorta diameter ratio greater than 1 should raise suspicion for pulmonary hypertension in intermediate-risk patients, including those with a prior history of acute pulmonary embolism.[5] An increased ratio of right ventricle (RV) to left ventricle (LV) transverse diameter greater than 1 with flattening of the interventricular septum

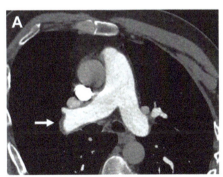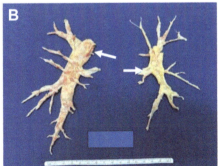

Fig. 4. Underestimation of disease extent on CTPA of a 72 year old man with CTEPH. (A) Preoperative CTPA demonstrated lining thrombus in the interlobar artery (arrow), but no conclusive disease in the main pulmonary arteries. (B) Surgical specimen following pulmonary thromboendarterectomy demonstrates lining thrombus in both main pulmonary arteries (arrows) in addition to the remainder of the pulmonary arterial tree.

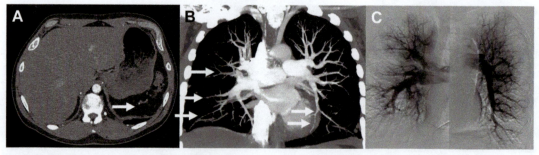

Fig. 5. Distal CTEPH in a 42 year old man with history of splenectomy in the setting of hereditary spherocytosis. (*A*) Axial image from CTPA through the upper abdomen demonstrates evidence of prior splenectomy. (*B*) Coronal MIP image demonstrates abnormal distal tapering of segmental and subsegmental pulmonary arteries, a typical pattern seen in postsplenectomy patients. (*C*) Anteroposterior images from digital subtraction angiography catheter angiography confirm evidence of segmental and subsegmental disease.

also suggests elevated right heart pressure. Thus, the finding of an elevated RV:LV ratio in a patient with acute pulmonary embolism can be equivocal for acute right heart strain in patients with underlying pulmonary hypertension. Right ventricular hypertrophy may be helpful for suggesting longstanding pulmonary hypertension, but the assessment can be difficult on a non-ECG-gated CT. Additionally, comparing current imaging with prior studies can also help determine chronicity of RV enlargement.

Preoperative Imaging

The first-line treatment of CTEPH is PTE. Suction thrombectomy is ineffective and potentially dangerous for chronic thromboembolism due to the strong adhesion of clots to the vessel wall. PTE involves removing the intimal lining of the pulmonary arteries along with the organized clot by dissecting along a plane in the media layer of the vessel wall. At experienced centers, it is possible to even remove disease at the subsegmental level through PTE, but expertise varies between institutions. Balloon pulmonary angioplasty (BPA) is a catheter-based technique used for patients who are not surgical candidates for PTE. BPA dilates stenotic or occluded vessels and may sometimes be combined with PTE. Finally, medical therapy employs various types of vasodilators, usually acting on smooth muscle cells, to alleviate pulmonary hypertension. Currently, riociguat is the only FDA-approved medication for inoperable or recurrent CTEPH, but medical therapy can be used in conjunction with PTE or BPA.

In addition to identifying CTEPH, radiologists can contribute to preprocedural planning through surgical classification. The University of California, San Diego (UCSD) surgical classification system assigns levels of disease based on the location of the most proximal thrombus in the right and left pulmonary arteries.[22] Level 1 involves the main pulmonary arteries, level 2 involves the lobar arteries, level 3 involves the segmental arteries, and level 4 involves the subsegmental arteries. Levels are assigned to both left and right sides. All levels of disease, including level 4 disease, can potentially be treated surgically at expert centers, but local surgical expertise, patient comorbidities, and degree of pulmonary hypertension may influence whether a patient is deemed operable. BPA is generally considered more suitable for level 3 and 4 disease.[23] Although CT can underestimate the extent of disease, it remains essential for determining surgical candidacy. Radiologists should describe the most proximal level of disease, with the understanding that surgical staging may reveal additional disease.

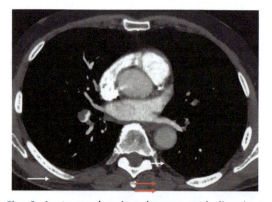

Fig. 6. Acute on chronic pulmonary embolism in a 73 year old man with acute dyspnea. Acute pulmonary embolism is present in the right lower lobe basal trunk and the inferior lingular pulmonary artery (*white arrows*). Note the convex borders of the right lower lobar pulmonary embolism and the expansile filling defect in the inferior lingular artery. The proximal left lower lobe segmental arteries (*red arrows*) are diminutive and contain webs, compatible with chronic thromboembolism.

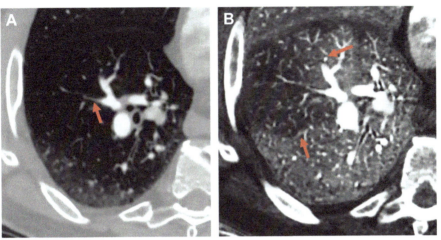

Fig. 7. Dual-energy CTPA of a 55 year old man with CTEPH. (*A*) Axial CTPA image demonstrates a diminutive subsegmental pulmonary artery in the right lower lobe anterior basal segment. (*B*) This abnormality is more apparent after observing a subsegmental perfusion defect on the corresponding iodine map, directing one's attention to the supplying pulmonary artery.

Additional findings on CT that may require concurrent repair during PTE include shunt lesions contributing to pulmonary hypertension, such as patent foramen ovale, atrial septal defect, or partial anomalous pulmonary venous return. Pulmonary hypertension can cause right-to-left flow through these lesions, resulting in an atypical appearance that may be easily missed. Chronic thrombus in the right atrium or ventricle should also be noted, as surgical removal may be required. This can be challenging to identify due to the mixing of opacified blood from the SVC and nonopacified blood from the inferior vena cava in the right atrium. Additionally, the presence of breast implants should be noted in patients undergoing minimally invasive PTE, as they may interfere with port placement. Finally, coronary artery disease, particularly in younger patients aged under 50 years, may prompt additional preoperative evaluation and possible revascularization.

Additional Modalities

Some institutions have explored the use of MR angiography for evaluating CTEPH, but its lower spatial resolution compared to CT reduces its sensitivity, particularly for detecting subsegmental disease.[24,25] However, MR offers several advantages, including the absence of ionizing radiation, the ability to assess pulmonary arterial flow, and detailed evaluation of the right ventricle.[26] MR perfusion techniques may perform similarly to

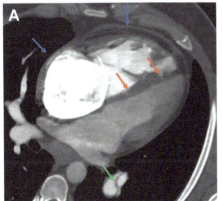
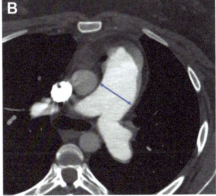

Fig. 8. CT findings of pulmonary hypertension. (*A*) Four chamber reformation from CT pulmonary angiogram demonstrates enlargement of the right atrium and right ventricle (*blue arrows*) with flattening of the interventricular septum (*red arrows*). The right ventricle is hypertrophied. Note the band in the left lower lobe basal trunk in this patient with CTEPH (*green arrow*). (*B*) Enlargement of the main pulmonary artery relative to the ascending aorta.

scintigraphy.[27] For now, MR imaging is generally considered an ancillary imaging modality rather than a primary one at most institutions, but its role may expand in the future.

Echocardiography, right heart catheterization, and catheter angiography are commonly performed in the CTEPH workup but are rarely interpreted by radiologists. Echocardiography remains the preferred noninvasive modality for the assessment of pulmonary hypertension in patients with persistent dyspnea following acute pulmonary embolism.[11] Right heart catheterization provides definitive hemodynamic characterization of pulmonary hypertension. Digital subtraction pulmonary angiography is commonly performed in the workup of CTEPH. In addition to demonstrating findings seen on CT such as pulmonary artery webs/bands, stenoses, and occlusions, it offers 2 key advantages: (1) it allows for better visualization of global vascular structure compared to CT pulmonary angiography, where overlapping pulmonary arteries and veins can make assessment challenging, and (2) it enables dynamic assessment of blood flow by showing vessel opacification over time.

DIAGNOSTIC CRITERIA

Diagnosis of CTEPH requires the identification of both CTEPD and pulmonary hypertension. CTEPD is typically identified through CT pulmonary angiography or catheter-based pulmonary angiography. While CT can suggest the presence of pulmonary hypertension, confirmation requires right heart catheterization. Pulmonary hypertension is defined as a mean pulmonary artery pressure greater than 20 mm Hg.[28] Patients with CTEPH specifically have precapillary hypertension, defined by a pulmonary artery wedge pressure of less than 15 mm Hg, and pulmonary vascular resistance of greater than 2 Wood units.

All CTEPH cases should be discussed by a multidisciplinary team consisting of pulmonologists, cardiothoracic surgeons, cardiologists, and radiologists to confirm the diagnosis and discuss treatment.[29,30] In some patients, CTEPD may contribute to pulmonary hypertension without being its primary cause, making it a less attractive target for treatment. In other cases, patients may have symptomatic CTEPD without resting pulmonary hypertension and could still benefit from treatment.

DIFFERENTIAL DIAGNOSIS

Conditions that can mimic CTEPH include acute pulmonary embolism, in situ thrombus, vasculitis, pulmonary artery sarcoma, and fibrosing mediastinitis. Acute pulmonary embolism was discussed earlier, and we will focus our discussion on the other entities. Although these conditions are relatively rare, it is important to recognize them, as their treatment differs significantly from that of CTEPH.

In Situ Thrombus

In situ thrombus refers to thrombus forming within the pulmonary arteries rather than embolizing from a deep vein. Similar to thrombus formation in other parts of the body, Virchow's triad of altered blood flow, endothelial injury, and hypercoagulability can lead to thrombus formation in the pulmonary arteries. For example, stump thrombus following pneumonectomy may result from endothelial injury and stasis of blood.

In the setting of CTEPH imaging, the most common differential consideration is pulmonary arterial hypertension with in situ thrombus, which can mimic CTEPH due to the presence of eccentric filling defects in the central pulmonary arteries (**Fig. 9**A–C).[31,32] However, extension of in situ thrombus into the segmental or subsegmental pulmonary arteries and vascular occlusions is rare, which typically distinguishes it from CTEPH. Additionally, in PAH, the "pruning" of pulmonary arteries tends to affect the entire arterial tree rather than specific areas corresponding to occluded vessels, a distinction often more evident when reviewing MIP images. Accordingly, mismatched defects on V/Q scan are generally smaller in patients with pulmonary arterial hypertension (PAH) and in situ thrombus, and hypoperfusion of the lung parenchyma generally involves smaller territories than those seen in CTEPH. Furthermore, PAH may demonstrate periarteriolar blushing,[33] which is atypical of CTEPH.

Other indirect findings can also help distinguish between PAH with in situ thrombus and CTEPH. Bronchial artery hypertrophy may be present in PAH but is generally less pronounced compared to CTEPH. Calcifications of the pulmonary arterial wall are uncommonly seen in CTEPH but occur in PAH due to significantly elevated pulmonary arterial pressure and development of atherosclerosis. However, calcification of thrombus itself is not useful for determining the underlying cause. Finally, infarcts and peripheral scarring are atypical in PAH.

Although in situ thrombus is more commonly seen in PAH, it can occur in any form of pulmonary hypertension (**Fig. 10**A, B), likely due to endothelial injury in the setting of high pressure. Interestingly, many patients with CTEPH have no history of deep vein thrombosis or acute pulmonary embolism,

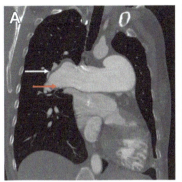 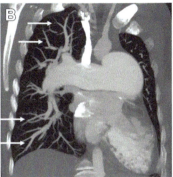 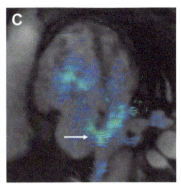

Fig. 9. A 43 year old man with in situ thrombus in the setting of unrepaired secundum atrial septal defect. (*A*) Coronal oblique image demonstrates massively dilated central pulmonary arteries. Lining thrombus is seen in the interlobar artery and proximal right upper lobe basal trunk (*white arrow*). Mural atherosclerotic calcification is present (*red arrow*), which is atypical of CTEPH. (*B*) Maximum intensity projection image from the same patient demonstrates patency of the distal segmental/subsegmental arteries, further confirming a non-CTEPH diagnosis. (*C*) A 4 chamber 4D flow MR image demonstrating marked enlarged of the right heart in keeping with pulmonary hypertension with right to left flow through the ASD in this still frame. Due to bidirectional flow, the pulmonary-to-systemic blood flow ratio (Qp/Qs) was 1.1.

suggesting that in situ thrombus could contribute to the pathophysiology of CTEPH.[34]

Pulmonary Artery Sarcoma

Intimal sarcoma of the pulmonary arteries is rare, but its imaging findings can overlap with those of CTEPH. Pulmonary artery sarcomas typically present as large filling defects in the central pulmonary arteries (**Fig. 11**A–C), with convex margins that often help distinguish them from chronic pulmonary embolism. Additional findings suggestive of a tumor include lung parenchymal or nodal metastatic disease, extravascular extension, or contrast enhancement.

However, there are cases where the imaging features of pulmonary artery sarcoma and CTEPH overlap. Pulmonary artery sarcomas may show concurrent bland thromboembolic disease, including occluded or diminished distal vessels and bronchial artery hypertrophy. While most central thrombus in CTEPH tends to be more peripheral, chronic or concurrent in situ thrombus can occasionally appear more space-occupying, complicating the differentiation.

PET-CT is reported to have a sensitivity of approximately 90%.[35] Alternatively, follow-up CT after 4 weeks may help identify enlarging filling defects, though care must be taken when assessing changes as bland thrombus may retract while tumor continues to grow. MR imaging may also be useful for identifying contrast enhancement, further aiding in the distinction between thrombus and tumor.

Vasculitis

Pulmonary arterial involvement of vasculitis has been described in large vessel vasculitis including Takayasu arteritis, giant cell arteritis, and Behçet disease (**Fig. 12**A–D). In most patients with

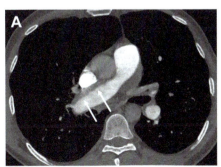 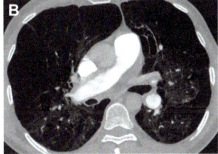

Fig. 10. A 55 year old man with in situ thrombus in the setting of smoking-related lung disease. (*A*) Axial CTPA image demonstrates lining thrombus of the right and interlobar pulmonary arteries. No thromboembolism was seen in segmental or subsegmental pulmonary arteries. (*B*) Corresponding lung windows demonstrate extensive centrilobular emphysema.

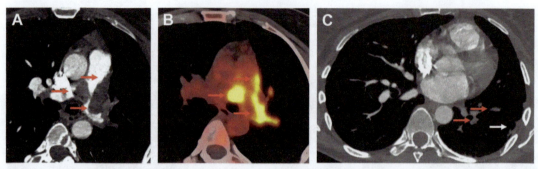

Fig. 11. A 43 year old woman with history of Lynch syndrome, dyspnea, and chest pain. (A) Axial oblique CTPA images demonstrate central pulmonary artery masses with convex margins which were initially interpreted as acute pulmonary embolism. (B) Subsequent PET-CT demonstrated heterogeneous fluorodeoxyglucose (FDG) uptake of the mass which may be due to admixed bland thrombus or non-FDG avid tumor. (C) Left lower lobe segmental arteries are occluded and diminutive (red arrows) relative to right-sided pulmonary arteries with associated infarct (white arrow), mimicking CTEPH. This may have been due to tumor, bland thrombus, or a combination of both.

Takayasu arteritis and giant cell arteritis, there will be concurrent evidence of systemic arterial involvement; however, in rare instances, pulmonary arterial involvement may occur in isolation. Overt wall thickening or enhancement is suggestive of arteritis, but other cases can mimic CTEPH with diminished vessel caliber and occluded distal pulmonary arteries. However, certain features can help distinguish vasculitis from CTEPH, such as the presence of "beading" in the pulmonary arteries, characterized by sequential stenosis and dilatation, which is atypical for CTEPH.

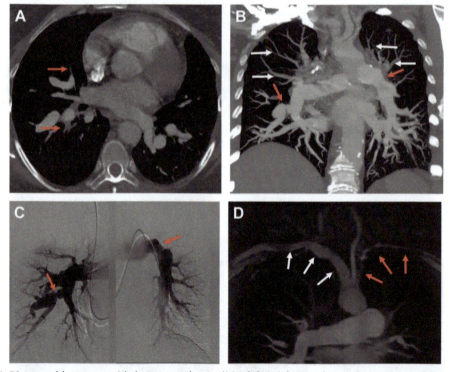

Fig. 12. A 59 year old woman with large vessel vasculitis. (A) Axial CT pulmonary angiogram image demonstrating diminutive medial segmental artery of the right middle lobe and proximal occlusion at the origin of the right lower lobe lateral and posterior basal segmental arteries (arrows). (B) Coronal oblique MIP image demonstrates unusual areas of vessel narrowing with beading of the anterior basal segmental artery of the right lower lobe and focal narrowing of the left descending pulmonary artery (red arrows). The upper lobe pulmonary arteries are occluded. These findings and distribution would be atypical of CTEPH and are more suggestive of vasculitis. (C) Digital subtraction angiography confirmed CT findings with redemonstrated areas of focal narrowing (arrows) and occluded upper lobe pulmonary arteries. (D) Subsequent MRA demonstrates segmental narrowing of the left axillosubclavian artery (red arrows) relative to the right axillosubclavian artery (white arrows).

Additionally, CTEPH shows greater involvement of the pulmonary arteries in the lower lobes, so predominant upper lobe involvement should raise suspicion for an alternative diagnosis.

Hughes–Stovin syndrome, which may represent a limited form of Behçet disease, is marked by focal pulmonary artery aneurysms or pseudoaneurysms. These aneurysms are usually more localized compared to the generalized arterial abnormalities seen in vasculitis affecting larger segments. Pulmonary artery aneurysms with lining thrombus are also uncommon in CTEPH.

Fibrosing Mediastinitis

Fibrosing mediastinitis is due to an exaggerated immune response to an antigen, most commonly from *Histoplasma capsulatum*. It is usually easy to distinguish from CTEPH, as pulmonary artery occlusions in fibrosing mediastinitis result from extrinsic compression by a mediastinal mass, rather than an intravascular process. Calcifications within the mediastinal mass are suggestive of a granulomatous origin, and splenic calcifications are often present.

Fibrosing mediastinitis more commonly affects the pulmonary veins, whereas CTEPH exclusively involves the pulmonary arteries. The distribution of pulmonary artery involvement in fibrosing mediastinitis can also differ from CTEPH. While CTEPH typically presents with bilateral, lower lung-predominant disease, fibrosing mediastinitis may show upper lobe predominance or unilateral involvement.

SUMMARY

CTEPH is an underdiagnosed but treatable condition, and radiologists play a critical role in improving patient care by recognizing CTED, particularly on CTPA. While chronic and acute pulmonary embolism have different imaging characteristics, distinguishing between the two can be challenging, especially when they coexist. Accurate imaging-based classification of CTEPH and identification of any additional pathology requiring surgical intervention are crucial in preoperative evaluation. Lastly, CTEPH has several mimics, but these conditions usually have distinct imaging features that help differentiate them.

CLINICS CARE POINTS

- The first-line screening for CTEPH is currently a V/Q scan, with SPECT-CT preferred when available.
- CT pulmonary angiography (CTPA) can be highly sensitive for detecting CTEPH, but the diagnosis is frequently missed by radiologists.
- Imaging findings of CTEPD differ from those of acute pulmonary embolism, though both chronic and acute disease may coexist on CTPA.
- Hypoperfusion can help pinpoint areas of CTEPD, a process that may be enhanced by spectral imaging techniques.
- Preoperative imaging aims to assess the extent of disease and identify other factors that could impact treatment decisions.
- Conditions that can mimic CTEPH include acute pulmonary embolism, in situ thrombus, pulmonary artery sarcoma, vasculitis, and fibrosing mediastinitis.

REFERENCES

1. Yan L, Li X, Liu Z, et al. Research progress on the pathogenesis of CTEPH. Heart Fail Rev 2019;24(6): 1031–40.
2. Madani MM. Pulmonary endarterectomy for chronic thromboembolic pulmonary hypertension: state-of-the-art 2020. Pulm Circ 2021;11(2). https://doi.org/10.1177/20458940211007372. 20458940211007372.
3. Guerin L, Couturaud F, Parent F, et al. Prevalence of chronic thromboembolic pulmonary hypertension after acute pulmonary embolism. Prevalence of CTEPH after pulmonary embolism. Thromb Haemost 2014;112(3):598–605.
4. Klok FA, Couturaud F, Delcroix M, et al. Diagnosis of chronic thromboembolic pulmonary hypertension after acute pulmonary embolism. Eur Respir J 2020; 55(6).
5. Remy-Jardin M, Ryerson CJ, Schiebler ML, et al. Imaging of pulmonary hypertension in adults: a position paper from the fleischner society. Radiology 2021;298(3):531–49.
6. Yang J, Madani MM, Mahmud E, et al. Evaluation and management of chronic thromboembolic pulmonary hypertension. Chest 2023;164(2):490–502.
7. Madani MM. Surgical treatment of chronic thromboembolic pulmonary hypertension: pulmonary thromboendarterectomy. Methodist Debakey Cardiovasc J 2016;12(4):213–8.
8. Auger WR, Kerr KM, Kim NH, et al. Evaluation of patients with chronic thromboembolic pulmonary hypertension for pulmonary endarterectomy. Pulm Circ 2012;2(2):155–62.
9. Wolf M, Boyer-Neumann C, Parent F, et al. Thrombotic risk factors in pulmonary hypertension. Eur Respir J 2000;15(2):395–9.

10. Simonneau G, Torbicki A, Dorfmuller P, et al. The pathophysiology of chronic thromboembolic pulmonary hypertension. Eur Respir Rev 2017;26(143). https://doi.org/10.1183/16000617.0112-2016.
11. Delcroix M, Torbicki A, Gopalan D, et al. ERS statement on chronic thromboembolic pulmonary hypertension. Eur Respir J 2021;57(6). https://doi.org/10.1183/13993003.02828-2020.
12. Michaud E, Pan M, Lakhter V, et al. Anatomical variations in pulmonary arterial branches in patients undergoing evaluation for chronic thromboembolic pulmonary hypertension. J Soc Cardiovasc Angiogr Interv 2023;2(5):101108.
13. Kandathil A, Chamarthy M. Pulmonary vascular anatomy & anatomical variants. Cardiovasc Diagn Ther 2018;8(3):201–7.
14. Cory RA, Valentine EJ. Varying patterns of the lobar branches of the pulmonary artery. A study of 524 lungs and lobes seen at operation of 426 patients. Thorax 1959;14(4):267–80.
15. Wittram C, Maher MM, Yoo AJ, et al. CT angiography of pulmonary embolism: diagnostic criteria and causes of misdiagnosis. Radiographics 2004;24(5):1219–38.
16. Fleischmann D. CT angiography: injection and acquisition technique. Radiol Clin North Am 2010;48(2):237–47, vii.
17. Bae KT. Intravenous contrast medium administration and scan timing at CT: considerations and approaches. Radiology 2010;256(1):32–61.
18. Patel S, Kazerooni EA. Helical CT for the evaluation of acute pulmonary embolism. AJR Am J Roentgenol 2005;185(1):135–49.
19. Wittram C. How I do it: CT pulmonary angiography. AJR Am J Roentgenol 2007;188(5):1255–61.
20. Hong YJ, Kim JY, Choe KO, et al. Different perfusion pattern between acute and chronic pulmonary thromboembolism: evaluation with two-phase dual-energy perfusion CT. AJR Am J Roentgenol 2013;200(4):812–7.
21. Poullis M. Thromboendarterectomy and circulatory arrest. Interact Cardiovasc Thorac Surg 2012;14(4):375–7.
22. Jenkins D, Madani M, Fadel E, et al. Pulmonary endarterectomy in the management of chronic thromboembolic pulmonary hypertension. Eur Respir Rev 2017;26(143). https://doi.org/10.1183/16000617.0111-2016.
23. Madani M, Ogo T, Simonneau G. The changing landscape of chronic thromboembolic pulmonary hypertension management. Eur Respir Rev 2017;26(146). https://doi.org/10.1183/16000617.0105-2017.
24. Ley S, Ley-Zaporozhan J, Pitton MB, et al. Diagnostic performance of state-of-the-art imaging techniques for morphological assessment of vascular abnormalities in patients with chronic thromboembolic pulmonary hypertension (CTEPH). Eur Radiol 2012;22(3):607–16.
25. Coulden R. State-of-the-art imaging techniques in chronic thromboembolic pulmonary hypertension. Proc Am Thorac Soc 2006;3(7):577–83.
26. Czerner CP, Schoenfeld C, Cebotari S, et al. Perioperative CTEPH patient monitoring with 2D phase-contrast MRI reflects clinical, cardiac and pulmonary perfusion changes after pulmonary endarterectomy. PLoS One 2020;15(9):e0238171.
27. Rajaram S, Swift AJ, Telfer A, et al. 3D contrast-enhanced lung perfusion MRI is an effective screening tool for chronic thromboembolic pulmonary hypertension: results from the ASPIRE Registry. Thorax 2013;68(7):677–8.
28. Humbert M, Kovacs G, Hoeper MM, et al, Group EESD. 2022 ESC/ERS Guidelines for the diagnosis and treatment of pulmonary hypertension. Eur Heart J 2022;43(38):3618–731.
29. Galie N, Humbert M, Vachiery JL, et al, Group ESCSD. 2015 ESC/ERS guidelines for the diagnosis and treatment of pulmonary hypertension: the joint task force for the diagnosis and treatment of pulmonary hypertension of the European society of cardiology (ESC) and the European respiratory society (ERS): endorsed by: association for European paediatric and congenital cardiology (AEPC), international society for heart and lung transplantation (ISHLT). Eur Heart J 2016;37(1):67–119.
30. Kim NH, Delcroix M, Jais X, et al. Chronic thromboembolic pulmonary hypertension. Eur Respir J 2019;53(1). https://doi.org/10.1183/13993003.01915-2018.
31. Agarwal PP, Wolfsohn AL, Matzinger FR, et al. In situ central pulmonary artery thrombosis in primary pulmonary hypertension. Acta Radiol 2005;46(7):696–700.
32. Hahn LD, Papamatheakis DG, Fernandes TM, et al. Multidisciplinary approach to chronic thromboembolic pulmonary hypertension: role of radiologists. Radiographics 2023;43(2):e220078.
33. Ridge CA, Bankier AA, Eisenberg RL. Mosaic attenuation. AJR Am J Roentgenol 2011;197(6):W970–7.
34. Baranga L, Khanuja S, Scott JA, et al. In situ pulmonary arterial thrombosis: literature review and clinical significance of a distinct entity. AJR Am J Roentgenol 2023;221(1):57–68.
35. Ropp AM, Burke AP, Kligerman SJ, et al. Intimal sarcoma of the great vessels. Radiographics 2021;41(2):361–79.

Imaging of Pulmonary Vasculitis

Donald Benson, MD, PhD

KEYWORDS

- Pulmonary vasculitis • Diffuse alveolar hemorrhage
- Antineutrophil cytoplasmic antibodies-associated vasculitis • Takayasu arteritis • Giant cell arteritis
- Behçet disease

KEY POINTS

- The pulmonary vasculitides are a heterogenous class of diseases that are associated with inflammation of the pulmonary blood vessel walls.
- Diffuse alveolar hemorrhage (DAH) is a common manifestation of pulmonary vasculitis and should be considered in patients with hemoptysis and imaging findings of diffuse ground-glass opacities or consolidation that do not improve with treatment for heart failure or infection.
- In evaluating patients with suspected pulmonary vasculitis, understanding the typical and atypical imaging appearances of common pulmonary vasculitides and reporting the pertinent positive and negative imaging findings can aid in diagnosis and classifying the patient using recent criteria.

INTRODUCTION
Introductory Case

A 38-year-old female with a history of rheumatoid arthritis arrived at the Emergency Department with acute chest pain. Her electrocardiographic findings were consistent with an anterior ST elevation myocardial infarct. She was emergently taken for catheter angiography, which showed 95% stenosis of the distal left anterior descending coronary artery and was treated with a stent. A computed tomography (CT) angiogram (CTA) of the neck, chest, abdomen, and pelvis at the time of admission showed focal thickening of the left subclavian artery causing severe stenosis along with multifocal narrowing and irregularity of the right vertebral artery (Fig. 1). These findings were not present on a neck CT performed 2 years earlier. Arterial wall thickening and narrowing of the bilateral iliac and femoral arteries were present and unchanged. Her initial blood work was significant for elevated erythrocyte segmentation rate and C-reactive protein.

The interpretation of the CTA of the neck favored atherosclerotic disease over vasculitis, while the CT angiogram of the chest, abdomen, and pelvis suggested vasculitis as the underlying cause. This study highlights the difficulty that can arise in assessing for vasculitis and the need to evaluate the complete clinical, radiologic, and often histologic pattern in patients with suspected vasculitis. This case will be discussed further in the concluding comments.

Background

The pulmonary vasculitides are a heterogenous class of diseases that are associated with inflammation of the pulmonary blood vessel walls. The different forms of vasculitis can be classified based on a variety of factors including pathogenesis, type of inflammation, distribution of organ involvement, and clinical manifestations. The 2012 Revised International Chapel Hill Consensus Conference Nomenclature of Vasculitides[1] provides the most frequently used system of nomenclature for the

---

Cardiopulmonary Imaging Section, Department of Radiology, University of Alabama at Birmingham, JTN 361, 619 19th Street South, Birmingham, AL 35294, USA
E-mail address: donaldbenson@uabmc.edu

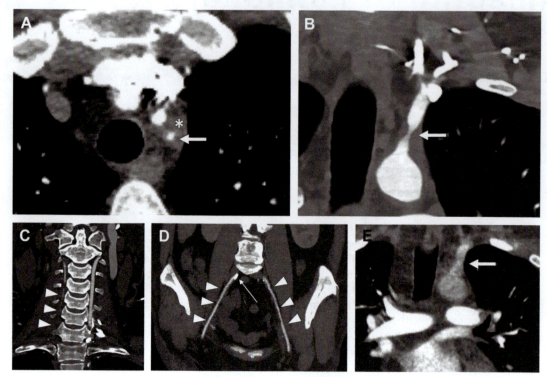

Fig. 1. Introductory Case: Axial (*A*) and Coronal (*B*) CT angiogram images with diffuse wall thickening of the left subclavian artery (*asterisk*) causing severe narrowing (*arrows*). Maximum intensity projection (MIP) coronal image (*C*) from the CT angiogram of the neck shows diffuse asymmetric multifocal narrowing of the right vertebral artery (*arrowheads*). (MIP) coronal image (*D*) from the CT angiogram of the pelvis shows vessel wall thickening and narrowing of the bilateral iliac arteries (*arrowheads*). Calcifications in the vessel walls are also present (*arrow*). A coronal image (*E*) from a pulmonary CT angiogram performed 3 months after the original CT shows decreased wall thickening and narrowing of the left subclavian artery (*arrow*).

various vasculitides. These diseases are first divided based on the size of the vessels that are most affected. Large vessel vasculitis (LVV) is primarily caused by inflammation of the aorta and its main branches. Medium vessel vasculitis (MVV) refers to inflammation of the arterial branches supplying major visceral organs like the kidneys. Small vessel vasculitis (SVV) involves the arterioles, capillaries, and venules. A few diseases have no predominant vessel involvement and fall under the category of variable vessel vasculitis (VVV). Many of the vasculitides are characterized by the presence of antineutrophil cytoplasmic antibodies (ANCA). Further classification can be made based on the distribution of organ involvement and clinical characteristics including age of onset.

In 2022, the American College of Rheumatology and the European Alliance of Associations for Rheumatology (ACR/EULAR) published new criteria for the classification of some of the large and small vessel vasculitides.[2–6] Several of these new criteria include imaging findings as part of the classification system, so it is important for radiologists to be aware of what findings need to be reported to aid in the classification of these disease processes. It is important to note that these criteria are used for disease classification and have not been validated solely for the diagnosis of any vasculitis. A diagnosis of a particular vasculitis should be based on all available clinical, radiologic, and pathologic information.

The purpose of this review is to give an overview of diseases that affect the pulmonary vasculature and to focus on the characteristic imaging findings associated with each type of vasculitis. This review will discuss some of the LVV and SVV. MVV, infectious vasculitis, vasculitis associated with systemic diseases (eg, rheumatoid arthritis and sarcoidosis), and vasculitis associated with probable etiologies (eg, cancer and hepatitis B and C) will not be discussed.

Pathophysiology

The pulmonary vasculitides are usually a manifestation of a broader systemic vasculitis, although they rarely can occur as a limited vasculitis confined to the respiratory system. Along with direct vessel wall inflammation, pulmonary involvement in vasculitis can occur through 3 mechanisms:

- Pulmonary capillaritis resulting in DAH
- Inflammatory cell infiltration of the lung parenchyma often resulting in necrosis or granuloma formation
- Inflammation of the tracheobronchial tree resulting in airway thickening, nodularity, stenosis, or some combination.

Most pulmonary vasculitides involve the smaller vessels, primarily capillaries. Involvement of the bronchial arteries and pulmonary arteries and veins can occur in LVV and VVV but is less common than involvement of the aorta and its larger branches.

The SVV are divided into immune complex and ANCA-associated vasculitides (AAV). In immune complex vasculitis, there is marked deposition of immune complexes in the affected vessel walls. In AAV, there is usually limited or no deposition of immune complexes in the vessel walls, and instead these diseases are characterized by the presence of antibodies directed against cytoplasmic components of neutrophils and monocytes.

Imaging Findings

Multiple imaging examinations are used in the assessment of pulmonary vasculitis. The advantages and disadvantages of each modality along with common imaging findings are discussed in **Table 1**.

Pathologically, pulmonary vasculitis most commonly affects the small pulmonary capillaries.[7] Capillaritis, the inflammation of pulmonary capillaries, leads to the destruction of the alveolar-capillary membrane allowing for alveolar leakage of red blood cells. The resulting DAH is one of the most common pulmonary manifestations of pulmonary vasculitis.

The classic radiologic appearance of DAH is bilateral ground-glass opacity (GGO) often with subpleural sparing (**Fig. 2**). Radiographs can be normal with DAH, making chest CT the imaging modality of choice. In the acute setting, diffuse GGO is often accompanied by interlobular septal thickening secondary to lymphatic congestion from hemosiderin laden macrophages resulting in a "crazy-paving" pattern.[8] The GGO can also coalesce into areas of consolidation (3). Consolidation can also be seen secondary to pulmonary infarcts. Organizing pneumonia near areas of hemorrhage resulting in a "reverse halo" can occur with some vasculitides.[9,10] Resolution of the radiologic abnormalities often lag behind the clinical resolution of symptoms. Granulomatous inflammation of the lung parenchyma commonly results in pulmonary nodules and masses, which can cavitate. Recurrent lung injury from repeated episodes of vasculitis can result in pulmonary fibrosis. Imaging is also important to exclude other potential causes of hemoptysis including bronchiectasis or malignancy.

Involvement of the upper and lower airways is common in many of the pulmonary vasculitides, and the pattern of airway involvement can help distinguish among different types of vasculitis. Upper airway involvement can lead to nasal obstruction and recurrent episodes of sinusitis. Repeated insults to the nasal passages can result in nasal septal destruction and collapse with saddle nose deformity. Oral ulcerations and gingival hyperplasia can also occur.

Acute and chronic airway inflammation from vasculitis can result in lower airway thickening and narrowing, most commonly involving the subglottic region (**Fig. 3**). Focal granulomatous inflammation can result in inflammatory nodules or pseudotumors. Tracheal webs and membranes can form. CT acquired at full inspiration can underestimate the degree of lower airway narrowing. Tracheobronchomalacia can also develop secondary to airway involvement of vasculitis. Therefore, CT acquisitions in full inspiration and expiration may be useful in the initial assessment of suspected pulmonary vasculitis.[11]

Vessel wall inflammation also occurs in MVV and LVV. On CT, the vascular abnormalities appear as vessel wall thickening, aneurysms, narrowing, and beading. MRI can add additional information with active inflammation characterized by increased signal on T2-weighted and short tau inversion recovery sequences and vessel wall enhancement on post-contrast T1-weighted sequences.

SMALL VESSEL VASCULITIDES
Antineutrophil Cytoplasmic Antibodies-associated Vasculitides

These diseases are associated with circulating antibodies against components found in the cytoplasm of neutrophils and monocytes. The presence of ANCA is useful in the diagnosis and classification of the 3 AAVs: granulomatosis with polyangiitis (GPA), microscopic polyangiitis (MPA), and eosinophilic granulomatosis with polyangiitis (EGPA). AAVs are the most common cause of pulmonary-renal syndrome consisting of both DAH and rapidly progressive glomerulonephritis. AAVs account for approximately 70% of patients with pulmonary-renal syndrome.[12] It is important to consider these diseases any time a patient presents with both lung abnormalities and renal impairment.

Table 1
Advantages, disadvantages and common imaging findings associated with common imaging modalities used in evaluating pulmonary vasculitis

Modality	Advantages	Disadvantages	Common Imaging Findings Seen in Pulmonary Vasculitis
Chest radiography	• Inexpensive, readily available • Low radiation exposure	• Limited sensitivity • Often underestimates overall disease burden	• Often normal • Diffuse or patchy bilateral lung opacities (see **Fig. 7**) • Multiple distinct lung nodules with cavitation occasionally present
Catheter angiography	• Can be used to treat aneurysms or active bleeding	• Invasive • Limited assessment of vessel wall	• Aneurysms • Vessel stenosis • Active bleeding
Ultrasound	• Inexpensive, readily available • No ionizing radiation exposure	• Operator dependent • Limited field of view	• Vessel wall thickening/edema "halo sign" (see **Fig. 12**) • Diminished Doppler flow • Vessel non-compressibility
Computed tomography (CT)	• Readily available • Rapid acquisition • High spatial resolution • Can simultaneously assess the lungs, airways, and vessels • Easily identifies calcifications	• Ionizing radiation exposure • Iodinated contrast administration contraindicated with severely impaired renal function	• Consolidation, ground-glass opacities, and nodules • Airway thickening and narrowing • Vessel wall thickening, aneurysms, and stenosis
Magnetic resonance imaging (MRI)	• Excellent contrast resolution for assessing subtle vessel wall inflammation • Fluid-weighted and contrast-enhanced images can detect active inflammation • No ionizing radiation	• Longer acquisition times • Challenging for claustrophobic patients given the small enclosed bore • Risk of nephrogenic sclerosing fibrosis in patients with impaired renal function (although these risks are significantly decreased with Group 2 and 3 agents[41]	• Vessel wall thickening and enhancement (see **Fig. 10**) • Aneurysms and stenosis • Perivascular inflammation
FDG- Positron emission tomography (PET)	• Expensive • Can combine functional imaging from PET with anatomic information from CT or MRI • Can be used for diagnosis and monitoring disease progression and assessment of response	• Ionizing radiation exposure • Longer acquisition times • Can be difficult to obtain in the acute setting	• Increased FDG uptake in areas of inflammation secondary to increased glucose metabolism from upregulation of glucose-tranporter-1 in activated inflammatory cells[42]

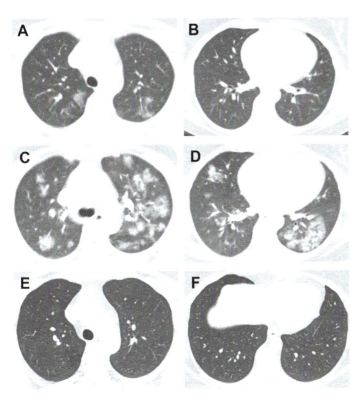

Fig. 2. Patient with MPA. 50-year-old female with unexplained iron deficiency anemia and hemoptysis. (*A* and *B*) Initial axial CT images with mild upper lung ground-glass opacities. (*C* and *D*). Axial CT images 1 month later with worsening ground-glass opacities throughout the lungs. She was found to p-ANCA positive with anti-MPO antibodies. Serial bronchial aliquots on bronchoscopy confirmed DAH. She was treated with rituximab and on subsequent CT, ground-glass opacities resolved, (*E* and *F*).

The presence of ANCA has been reported in up to 96% of GPA patients with severe disease and 83% in limited disease with most ANCA-positive patients reactive to c-ANCA/PR3-ANCA.[13] Up to 75% of patients with MPA are ANCA positive,[13] the majority of which are perinuclear (p)-ANCA/ myeloperoxidase (MPO)-ANCA reactive.[14] With EGPA, ANCAs are detected in approximately half of patients with the majority of those reactive to p-ANCA/MPO-ANCA.[15]

Granulomatosis with polyangiitis

GPA, referred to as Wegener granulomatosis until 2011,[16] is the most common of the AAVs, although incidence and prevalence among the AAVs has considerable geographic variation.[17,18] GPA equally effects men and women.[19] The classic clinical triad includes upper airway involvement, lower respiratory involvement, and glomerulonephritis. However, GPA can involve multiple other organs including the skin, eyes, heart, nervous system, muscles, and joints.[20] Histologically, GPA is characterized by extravascular granulomatous inflammation along with necrotizing vasculitis affecting small and medium sized vessels leading to vascular thrombosis and tissue necrosis.[21,22] Most patients respond well to treatment, which typically involves an induction phase using immunosuppressive drugs, commonly cyclophosphamide, with or without corticosteroids, followed by long-term immunosuppressive maintenance therapy for disease remission.[23]

The characteristic radiographic abnormality in GPA patients with active disease is multiple pulmonary nodules and masses, which often cavitate (**Fig. 4**). CT is the preferred imaging modality for the detection of cavitary and noncavitary nodules.

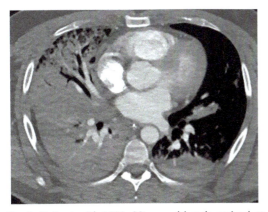

Fig. 3. Patient with MPA. 32-year-old male arrived at the Emergency Department with hemoptysis and was found to have renal failure. Axial CT image of the chest at that time showed diffuse consolidation, and DAH was confirmed on bronchoscopy. He was later found to have anti-MPO antibodies.

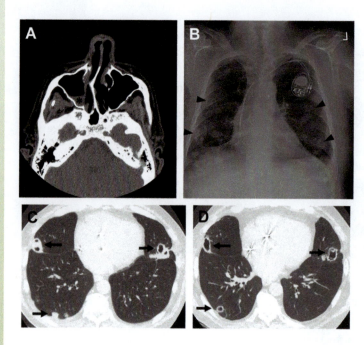

Fig. 4. Patient with GPA. A 79-year-old male came to the Emergency Department with shortness of breath and symptoms of sinusitis. (*A*) Axial sinus CT image showed an air-fluid level in the right maxillary sinus (*asterisk*) consistent with acute sinusitis. (*B*) Chest radiograph at that time demonstrated multiple bilateral cavitary nodules (*arrowheads*). (*C*) On the chest CT, there were multiple solid and cavitary lung nodules (*arrows*). He was found to be c-ANCA positive with anti-PR3 antibodies. (*D*) After treatment, the cavitary nodules (*arrows*) improved with decreased thickness of the cavity walls.

One study of 30 patients found nodules in approximately 90% of patients at initial presentation.[24] In this study, 85% of patients had multiple nodules with bilateral nodules in 67% of patients. These nodules favored subpleural predominance over a peribronchovascular distribution. The nodules often coalesce and can often be secondarily infected. The halo sign can be seen secondary to hemorrhage adjacent to nodules in up to 15% of patients.[24] An organizing pneumonia pattern of lung injury has been reported in GPA[9] GGO and consolidation can also occur in the setting of active vasculitis and capillaritis leading to DAH.

Airway involvement is reported in up to 60% to 70% of patients with GPA[20,25] with tracheal involvement in 30% of patients. The subglottic trachea is the most common site with tracheal wall thickening, nodularity, and stenosis reported (**Fig. 5**). In a study of 962 patients,[26] 10% of patients had subglottic stenosis, and 6% of patients had endobronchial disease. Involvement of the posterior membrane is common in patients with GPA,[27] helping to distinguish it from relapsing polychondritis.

The 2022 ACR/EULAR classification criteria for GPA[5] is applied to patients with a diagnosis of SVV or MVV and suspicion for GPA (**Fig. 6**). This classification utilizes a scoring system involving clinical, laboratory, imaging, and biopsy criteria. The relevant imaging findings are discussed in **Box 1**.

Microscopic polyangiitis
MPA is also a pauci-immune necrotizing vasculitis; however, unlike with GPA, granulomatous inflammation is absent. While MPA can affect medium sized vessels, it is predominantly a small-vessel vasculitis resulting in glomerulonephritis and pulmonary capillaritis. MPA is a common cause of pulmonary-renal syndrome with renal involvement occurring in more than 90% of patients. Many patients have a prodromal syndrome of fever and weight loss occurring prior to the development of rapidly progressing glomerulonephritis.

Pulmonary involvement is less common than renal involvement, occurring in only 30% of patients. The primary imaging finding is DAH secondary to pulmonary capillaritis (see **Fig. 2**). As described earlier, radiographs of patients with DAH can be normal or show diffuse opacities. CT shows GGO and consolidation, which are commonly bilateral and can be patchy or diffuse (see **Fig. 3**). These are usually perihilar with subpleural sparing. Repeated pulmonary insults can lead to pulmonary fibrosis, which is more common with MPA than GPA and often has a poor prognosis.

The relevant imaging findings from the 2022 ACR/EULAR classification criteria for MPA[6] are summarized in **Box 2**.

Eosinophilic granulomatosis with polyangiitis
Eosinophilic granulomatosis with polyangiitis (EGPA), renamed from Churg-Strauss syndrome in the 2012 Chapel Hill classification, is a rare disease characterized by asthma, peripheral eosinophilia, and necrotizing vasculitis. Lung involvement is common with asthma occurring in almost all (91%–100%)[28] of patients with EGPA. Cardiac abnormalities occur in 13% to 47% of patients[29] and are a leading cause of mortality. Other organs

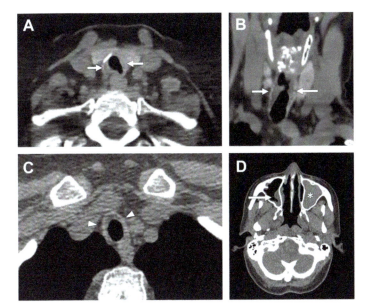

Fig. 5. Tracheal disease in GPA. Patient 1 - 60-year-old female with shortness of breath and c-ANCA positive. She had no imaging abnormalities in her sinuses or lungs but did have focal subglottic narrowing of the trachea here on axial (A) and coronal (B) CT images (arrows). Patient 2 to 57-year-old female with recurrent sinusitis and found to have anti-PR3 antibodies. (C) Axial CT showed focal thickening (arrowhead) of the upper thoracic trachea. (D) Axial sinus CT image with complete opacification of the left maxillary sinus (asterisk) and polypoid mucosal thickening in the right maxillary sinus (arrow).

involved include the skin, gastrointestinal (GI) tract, and kidneys. Peripheral neuropathy is common affecting up to 75% of patients.

Many patients are often p-ANCA or anti-MPO positive, although this is less common than in the other AAV. Glomerulonephritis is also less common, although almost all EGPA patients with glomerulonephritis show ANCA-positivity.[30] In fact, most patients with vasculitic signs symptoms including glomerulonephritis, purpura, and peripheral neuropathy are more commonly ANCA positive, while those with eosinophilic predominant features including gastroenteritis and cardiac involvement tend to be ANCA-negative.[31]

The characteristic findings in patients with EGPA on chest radiographs are multiple areas of consolidation that tend to be peripheral (Fig. 7). The most common findings on CT are bilateral areas of GGO and consolidation that tend to be peripheral and lower lung predominant, similar to eosinophilic pneumonia (Fig. 8). These are commonly transient. Interlobular septal thickening may be present due to eosinophilic lymphatic infiltrates or from pulmonary edema in patients with cardiac involvement. Pleural effusions can also occur in patients with cardiomyopathy or eosinophilic pleuritis.

Large and small airway involvement is commonly present in patients with EGPA. Bronchial wall thickening can occur secondary to eosinophilic infiltrates in the airway walls (see Fig. 8). Small centrilobular nodules are secondary to eosinophilic bronchiolitis. It is important to highlight the difference between airway predominant disease and airspace predominant disease in patients with EGPA since patients with airspace predominant disease may respond better to treatment.[32]

Cardiac involvement can be occur with hypereosinophilia and is responsible for up to half of EGPA-related deaths.[33] Cardiac disease is the result of eosinophilic infiltration of the myocardium resulting in cardiomyopathy and diastolic dysfunction. Intracardiac thrombus is a common. Cardiac MRI is the imaging modality of choice with active myocardial inflammation identifiable on T2-weighted images, while delayed-gadolinium enhanced images show the subendocardial fibrosis (Fig. 9) and nonenhancing mural thrombus.

The 2022 ACR/EULAR classification criteria for EGPA[2] are summarized in Box 3.

Immune Complex Small Vessel Vasculitis

Many immune mediated processes can result in the deposition of immunoglobulin or complement in the vessel walls. These processes frequently involve many organ systems with glomerulonephritis occurring in most patients. Pulmonary involvement is usually less common than in the pauci-immune small vessel vasculitides with DAH being the most common manifestation. Imaging findings alone are unlikely to lead to a diagnosis in these conditions, but when presented with a patient with suspicion for one of these conditions, it is important to be aware of the expected imaging findings. A few of these vasculitides with pulmonary involvement are described in Table 2.

2022 AMERICAN COLLEGE OF RHEUMATOLOGY / EUROPEAN ALLIANCE OF ASSOCIATIONS FOR RHEUMATOLOGY CLASSIFICATION CRITERIA FOR GRANULOMATOSIS WITH POLYANGIITIS

CONSIDERATIONS WHEN APPLYING THESE CRITERIA
- These classification criteria should be applied to classify a patient as having granulomatosis with polyangiitis when a diagnosis of small- or medium-vessel vasculitis has been made
- Alternate diagnoses mimicking vasculitis should be excluded prior to applying the criteria

CLINICAL CRITERIA

Nasal involvement: bloody discharge, ulcers, crusting, congestion, blockage, or septal defect/perforation	+3
Cartilaginous involvement (inflammation of ear or nose cartilage, hoarse voice or stridor, endobronchial involvement, or saddle nose deformity)	+2
Conductive or sensorineural hearing loss	+1

LABORATORY, IMAGING, AND BIOPSY CRITERIA

Positive test for cytoplasmic antineutrophil cytoplasmic antibodies (cANCA) or antiproteinase 3 (anti-PR3) antibodies	+5
Pulmonary nodules, mass, or cavitation on chest imaging	+2
Granuloma, extravascular granulomatous inflammation, or giant cells on biopsy	+2
Inflammation, consolidation, or effusion of the nasal/paranasal sinuses, or mastoiditis on imaging	+1
Pauci-immune glomerulonephritis on biopsy	+1
Positive test for perinuclear antineutrophil cytoplasmic antibodies (pANCA) or antimyeloperoxidase (anti-MPO) antibodies	-1
Blood eosinophil count ≥ 1 x10⁹/liter	-4

Sum the scores for 10 items, if present. A score of ≥ 5 is needed for classification of GRANULOMATOSIS WITH POLYANGIITIS.

Fig. 6. 2022 American College of Rheumatology/European Alliance of Associations for Rheumatology classification criteria for granulomatosis with polyangiitis. (*From* Robson JC, Grayson PC, Ponte C, et al. 2022 American College of Rheumatology/European Alliance of Associations for Rheumatology Classification Criteria for Granulomatosis With Polyangiitis. Arthritis & Rheumatology. 2022;74(3):393 to 399. doi:https://doi.org/10.1002/art.41986.)

LARGE VESSEL VASCULITIDES

According to the 2012 Chapel Hill Classification, LVV can involve vessels of all sizes but more commonly affect the large vessels than other vasculitides.[1] In some patients, the medium and small vessels may be more affected than the large vessels. There are 2 major LVV, Takayasu arteritis (TAK) and giant cell arteritis (GCA), which appear similar on histopathology with some suggesting that they may be the same processes. Historically, they have been separated based on age of onset and the distribution of vascular involvement.

Box 1
Summary of the 2022 ACR/EULAR classification criteria for GPA[5]

- A score of greater than or equal to 5 is required.
- Important imaging findings to report:
  - Pulmonary nodules, mass or cavitation - 2 points
  - Nasal/paranasal sinus inflammation or mastoiditis - 1 point
  - Cartilaginous involvement (tracheobronchial thickening/nodularity or ear or nasal cartilage inflammation/deformity) – 2 points.

Box 2
Summary of the 2022 ACR/EULAR classification criteria for MPA[6]

- A score of greater than or equal to 5 is required.
- The presence of fibrosis adds 3 points.
- Nasal involvement on clinical assessment or imaging will decrease the score by 3 as this is not commonly seen with MPA.

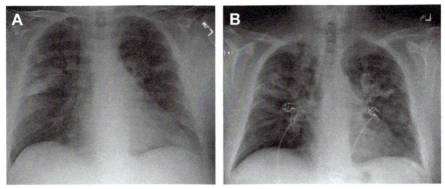

Fig. 7. (A) Anterior-posterior chest radiograph of a patient with eosinophilic granulomatosis with polyangiitis shows patchy multifocal areas of consolidation. (B) Posterior-anterior radiograph 2 weeks later shows improvement in the right upper lobe consolidation with new areas of peribronchovascular consolidation bilaterally and increased nodularity.

Takayasu Arteritis

TAK was first described by Dr Takayasu over 100 years ago in a report of a patient with abnormalities of the retinal vessels.[34] TAK most commonly involves the aorta and its branches and has classically been described in females from East Asia, although this disease is now known to affect patients worldwide and can also affect males. TAK most frequently affects patients under the age of 40 year old. This disease is the result of granulomatous inflammation primarily involving the large and small vessels. Chronic inflammation leads to segmental vessel wall thickening, stenosis, and thrombosis.

Chest radiography is often normal. However, occasionally dilation of the thoracic aorta or of the arch vessels can result in mediastinal widening. Ultrasound is usually not often helpful since most

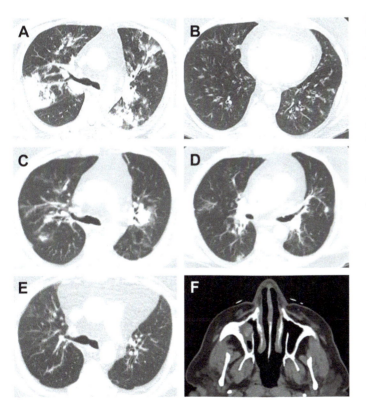

Fig. 8. Patient with EGPA. 33-year-old male with a history of recurrent asthma and chronic papular skin rash presented with concern for pneumonia and painless right vision loss. Initial CT images of the chest showed (A) patchy areas of peripheral and peribronchial consolidation in the upper lobes and (B) bronchial wall thickening and peribronchial ground-glass opacities in the lower lungs. He was found to have central retinal arterial occlusion and peripheral eosinophilia with AEC of 15,000/mm^3. A biopsy of the papular rash showed small vessel vasculitis (SVV) with eosinophils and granuloma formation. On the CT a few days later, (C) right upper lobe consolidation improved, but there was new left perihilar consolidation. (D) Lung nodules alos developed. He was started on steroids and cyclophosphamide. After treatment, most of the lung abnormalities resolved with some residual reticulation and ground-glass opacities on on CT 1 year later (E). (F) At initial presentation, sinus CT showed surgical changes of both maxillary sinuses with partial calcified soft tissue density in the right maxillary sinus suggestive of chronic fungal infection.

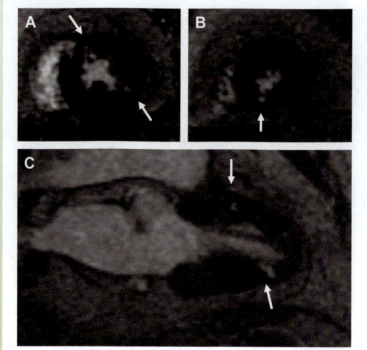

Fig. 9. Cardiac MRI of the patient with EGPA in Fig. 8. Short axis (*A* and *B*) and two-chamber (*C*) late gadolinium enhanced images show multifocal areas of mid-myocardial delayed enhancement involving the anterior and inferolateral walls in the mid segment (*A*) and in the inferior wall in the distal segment (*B*), suggesting focal areas of myocardial fibrosis.

of the involved vessels are not accessible. CT and MRI are the imaging modalities of choice, with both able to clearly show areas of vessel wall thickening and stenosis. MRI can also show areas of active inflammation on T2-weighted and gadolinium enhanced imaging (**Fig. 10**). Fludeoxyglucose-18 (FDG)-PET can also evaluate for active inflammation and can be used to assess for treatment response (**Fig. 11**).

Although aortic involvement is most common, patients with TAK can also have abnormalities of the pulmonary arteries with wall thickening and active inflammation in the larger pulmonary arteries.[35] In the segmental and subsegmental pulmonary arteries, areas of focal stenosis or occlusion can develop, resulting in decreased perfusion on MRI or on the iodine maps of dual energy CT similar to pulmonary embolism. With chronic disease, calcifications can form in the pulmonary artery walls. Collateralization of bronchial or intercostal arteries can also occur with chronic disease.[35]

All patients with suspected TAK are recommended for evaluation with magnetic resonance angiography (MRA), CTA, or FDG-PET.[36] Given the younger patient population, MRA is the first line imaging modality recommended due to the lack of ionizing radiation.

The relevant imaging findings from the 2022 ACR/EULAR classification criteria for TAK[3] are discussed in **Box 4**.

Giant Cell Arteritis

GCA is also an LVV primarily affecting the aorta and its branches and, like TAK, is characterized histologically by granulomatous inflammation of the vessel walls. GCA commonly affects the cranial branches of the carotid and vertebral arteries. GCA typically presents at a later age than TAK with most GCA patients presenting after the age of 50 years. Another distinguishing factor between GCA and TAK is that involvement of the temporal artery is more common with GCA with up to 60% of temporal artery biopsies in patient with GCA showing granulomatous inflammation. However, temporal artery involvement is not diagnostic for

---

Box 3
Summary of the 2022 ACR/EULAR classification criteria for EGPA[2]

- A score of greater than or equal to 6 is required.
- No direct imaging findings are included.
- The clinical presence of obstructive airway disease adds 3, so it is important to point out air-trapping when present.
- The presence of nasal polyps adds 3 points, so it is important to assess for this if imaging of the nasal passages is available.

Table 2
Description of immune complex vasculitides with pulmonary involvement

Vasculitis	Pathogenesis	Clinical Presentation	Pulmonary Imaging Findings
Hypocomplementemic urticarial (anti-C1q) vasculitis	• Hypocomplementemia from destruction of complement secondary to excess anti-C1q antibodies • Increased elastase release from neutrophils resulting in alveolar destruction	• COPD or asthma • Urticaria, glomerulonephritis, arthritis, and ocular involvement	• Emphysema, often lower lung panlobular
Immunoglobulin A vasculitis (Henoch-Schönlein purpura)	• IgA1 deposition in vessel walls	• Most frequently occurs in children • Often preceded by respiratory or GI illness • Purpureal rash common • Can also involve kidneys, GI tract, and joints	• DAH can occur in adults, rare in children • Pulmonary fibrosis can occur secondary to severe or recurrent disease
Anti-glomerular basement membrane (anti-GBM) disease (Goodpasture disease)	• Circulating antibodies interact with antigens on the glomerular and alveolar basement membranes	• Glomerulonephritis occurs almost universally • Pulmonary involvement less common (40%–50%)	• DAH secondary to pulmonary capillaritis

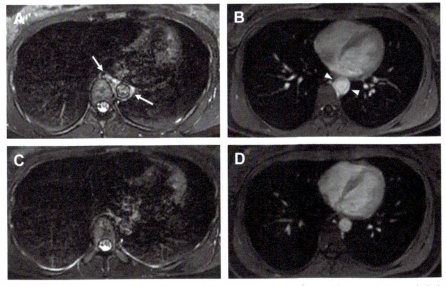

Fig. 10. Patient with Takayasu arteritis. A 26-year-old female came to clinic with several days of abdominal and chest pain. Her blood work was significant for elevated ESR and CRP levels. (*A*) Axial T2-weighted short-tau inversion recovery MRI images showed increase T2 signal surrounding the descending thoracic aorta (*arrows*). (*B*) Contrast enhanced axial T1-weighted MRI images also showed enhancing circumferential wall thickening (*arrowheads*) of the descending thoracic aorta consistent with active arteritis. Her symptoms improved after she was placed on methotrexate and prednisone. (*C* and *D*) MRI images obtained approximately 1 year later show resolution of the previous abnormalities.

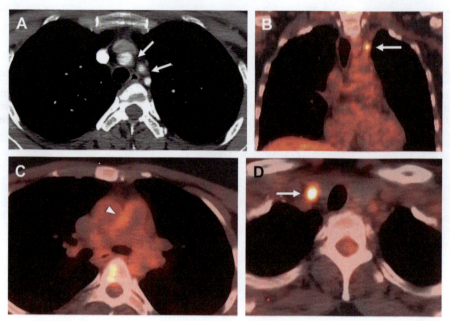

Fig. 11. Another patient with Takayasu arteritis. (*A*). Axial CT of the chest with soft tissue thickening (*arrows*) of the right brachiocephalic and left common carotid arteries. (*B*) Coronal fused PET/CT image with intense FDG uptake in the left common carotid artery (*arrow*). (*C* and *D*) Axial fused PET/CT images show increased FDG uptake between the ascending aorta and pulmonary trunk (*arrowhead*) and in the right common carotid artery (*arrow*).

GCA given that temporal artery involvement occurs with other forms of vasculitis and many patients with GCA lack involvement of the temporal artery.

Patients with cranial GCA commonly present with fever, headache, jaw pain, and vision disturbances. Ophthalmic involvement can lead to blindness and is considered an emergency requiring prompt treatment with high-dose steroids. While cranial involvement is the hallmark of GCA, extracranial involvement of the aorta and its extracranial branches occurs in 80% of patients. Thoracic aortic aneurysms are more common in patients with GCA compared to the general population, and dissection has been reported in 6% of patients with GCA.

Ultrasound is becoming more widely used in the diagnosis of GCA with the presence of vessel wall edema in the temporal artery characterized by hypoechoic, noncompressible vessel wall thickening (**Fig. 12**) considered a strong predictor of GCA. In Europe, recent guidelines[37] recommend the use of temporal artery ultrasound as the first line imaging test for GCA. However, given the lack of experience with temporal artery ultrasound in the United States, temporal artery biopsy remains the preferred initial diagnostic test in based societal guidelines.[36]

The imaging findings on CT and MRI are like those of TAK including vessel wall thickening, stenosis, and thrombosis. Involvement of the brachiocephalic, subclavian, and femoral arteries is common with large vessel GCA. Pulmonary artery involvement is less common than with TAK. FDG-PET

Box 4
Summary of the 2022 ACR/EULAR classification criteria for Takayasu arteritis[3]

Requirements:

- Diagnosis of large or MVV
- Imaging findings of vasculitis in the aorta or branch vessels by angiography (CT, MRI, or catheter directed) or PET
- Age 60 or less at the time of diagnosis
- A score of 5 or greater.

Imaging findings (vessel lumen damage defined by stenosis, occlusion, or aneurysm):

- Abdominal aortic involvement with renal or mesenteric involvement – 3 points
- Involvement of one or more of the following nine territories: thoracic aorta, abdominal aorta, mesenteric, left or right carotid, left or right subclavian, left or right renal - 1 point for one territory, 2 points for two territories or 3 points for three or more territories.
- Symmetric involvement of the paired carotid, subclavian or renal arteries - 2 points

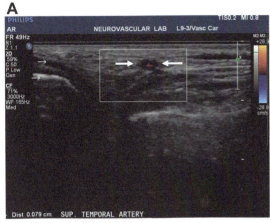 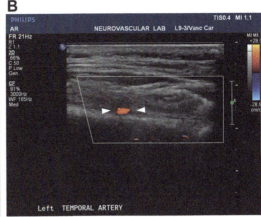

Fig. 12. (A) Doppler ultrasound of an abnormal left temporal artery (*arrows*) in a patient with GCA shows a dark ring ("halo sign") around the periphery of the artery with diminished flow. (B) Doppler ultrasound of a normal temporal artery (*arrowheads*) without the halo sign and normal Doppler flow.

can also be used to evaluate for active inflammation in patients with GCA, but assessment is less straightforward given the older patient population and increase in atherosclerotic disease.

The 2022 ACR/EULAR classification criteria for GCA[4] include several relevant imaging findings.(see **Box 5**).

Variable Vessel Vasculitides

Behçet disease is the most common cause of pulmonary artery aneurysms, which are rare. Clinically, Behçet disease is characterized by oral and genital ulcers although involvement of the eyes, joints, GI tract, and central nervous system are common.

Vascular involvement with Behçet disease only occurs in 25% to 30% of patients with venous abnormalities more common than arterial.[38] Thrombophlebitis is the most common venous abnormality, and venous occlusions occur most commonly in the superior vena cava, potentially leading to superior vena cava syndrome. Arterial involvement more commonly results in aneurysms than occlusions with the aorta more frequently involved than the pulmonary arteries. Pulmonary involvement is quite uncommon affecting only up to 8% of patients.[39] Patients typically present with cough, dyspnea, chest pain, and hemoptysis. The classic pulmonary imaging finding associated with Behçet disease are multiple bilateral pulmonary artery fusiform or saccular aneurysms. Other common findings include varices, pulmonary thromboembolism, and pulmonary infarctions.

The most common findings of Behçet disease on chest radiographs are peripheral areas of consolidation from pulmonary infarcts or multifocal areas of consolidation secondary to pulmonary hemorrhage.

Pulmonary artery aneurysms may be too small to be detected on chest radiographs, but larger aneurysms can appear as lung nodules or masses. Central pulmonary artery aneurysms can result in hilar or mediastinal widening. These findings are better demonstrated on CT or MRI, which are superior for assessing the size and distribution of pulmonary artery aneurysms and for evaluating for thrombus (**Fig. 13**). Perivascular inflammation can result in wall thickening. T2-weighted and gadolinium enhanced MRI sequences are used to assess for active inflammation.

Some aneurysms are responsive to immunosuppressive therapies with resolution reported in some patients.[40] However, there is a high risk of rupture if untreated. Parenchymal abnormalities adjacent to the aneurysms should raise concern

---

Box 5
Summary of the 2022 ACR/EULAR classification criteria for giant cell arteritis[4]

- A score of greater than or equal to 6 in a patient aged 50 or older is required.
- Important imaging findings to report:
  - Presence of a halo sign on temporal artery ultrasound (equivalent to a positive temporal artery biopsy) - 5 points
  - FDG uptake greater than liver uptake in the arterial wall of the descending thoracic aorta and/or abdominal aorta - 2 points.
  - Bilateral axillary arterial involvement characterized by stenosis, occlusion or aneurysm on ultrasound or angiography (CT, MR, or catheter), halo sign on ultrasound, or increased FDG uptake - 2 points.

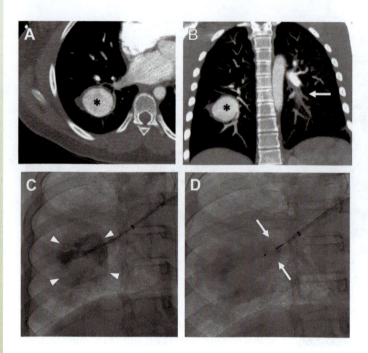

Fig. 13. Behçet disease. A 14-year-old female with a history of a resected cardiac mass (organized thrombus) came to the Emergency Department with hemoptysis and shortness of breath. (A) Axial pulmonary CTA shows a large aneurysm (asterisk) of a right lower lobe segmental pulmonary artery. (B) Coronal maximum intensity projection (MIP) images also show left lower lobe pulmonary embolism (arrow). (C) Catheter angiogram shows the large aneurysm (arrowheads). Embolization with an Amplatzer device (arrows) was performed (D). Unfortunately, the embolization was unsuccessful, and the patient underwent right lower lobectomy.

for impending rupture (Fig. 14). Mural calcifications can develop with long-standing disease.

Hughes-Stovin syndrome is believed to be a limited presentation of Behçet disease without the presence of oral or genital ulceration. Typically, patients have multiple pulmonary artery aneurysms and pulmonary arterial and venous occlusions or thrombi (see Fig. 14).

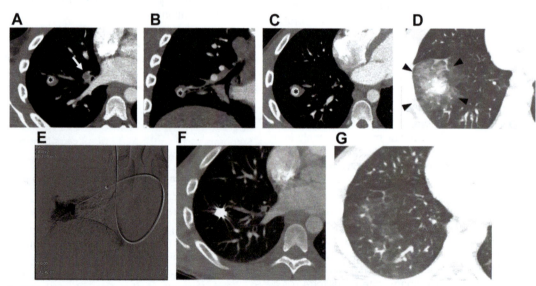

Fig. 14. A 23-year-old-male was admitted to the hospital for fevers, chills, and hemoptysis. Axial (A) and coronal (B) CT pulmonary angiogram images show pulmonary artery aneurysms (asterisks) and filling defects (arrow). Axial images in soft tissue window (C) and lung window settings (D) from a subsequent CT pulmonary angiogram show enlargement of the right lower lobe pulmonary artery aneurysm (asterisk) with new adjacent hemorrhage (arrowheads) suggesting impending rupture. Subsequent catheter angiogram (E) and embolization were performed. Subsequent chest CT shows the treated aneurysm (F) and axial lung window image shows resolution of hemorrhage adjacent to the aneurysm (G). This patient had no oral or genital ulcers and was diagnosed with Hughes-Stovin syndrome.

SUMMARY
Introductory Case Revisited

Rheumatology was consulted to assess the patient in the introductory case. Based on the clinical presentation and radiologic findings, active vasculitis was favored over atherosclerotic disease as the cause of the vascular abnormalities. Given the patient's age and sex, TAK was suspected, and she was started on steroids and methotrexate. Repeat imaging 3 month later showed decreased vessel wall thickening and reduced narrowing of the left subclavian artery, further supporting the diagnosis of vasculitis. This case demonstrates the importance of having a high clinical suspicion for vasculitis in patients with abnormal clinical and imaging findings that cannot be explained by other etiologies.

SUMMARY

Diagnosing pulmonary vasculitis can be challenging given that clinical signs and symptoms are vague and imaging findings are nonspecific and often overlap with other diseases. The introductory case demonstrates the importance of having a high clinical suspicion for vasculitis in patients with abnormal clinical and imaging findings that cannot be explained by other etiologies. A multidisciplinary approach to these complex patients can result in rapid diagnosis and treatment. Radiologists need to be aware of the common clinical and imaging findings associated with the vasculitides discussed and recognize the important imaging findings to highlight in order to assist in making the correct diagnosis.

CLINICS CARE POINTS

- Diagnosis of pulmonary vasculitis can be challenging and requires a high level of clinical suspicion and knowledge of relevant clinical, pathologic, and radiologic findings.
- Diagnostic criteria for these diseases are constantly evolving, and it is important for radiologists to be aware of the relevant imaging findings in recent classification criteria.

ACKNOWLEDGMENTS

The author would like to acknowledge Nina Terry, MD, JD and Padma Manapragada, MD for contributing cases and for editing and improving the article.

DISCLOSURE

The author has nothing to disclose.

REFERENCES

1. Jennette JC, Falk RJ, Bacon PA, et al. 2012 revised International Chapel Hill Consensus Conference Nomenclature of Vasculitides. Arthritis Rheum 2013; 65(1):1–11.
2. Grayson PC, Ponte C, Suppiah R, et al. American College of Rheumatology/European Alliance of Associations for Rheumatology Classification Criteria for Eosinophilic Granulomatosis With Polyangiitis. Arthritis Rheumatol 2022;74(3):386–92.
3. Grayson PC, Ponte C, Suppiah R, et al. American College of Rheumatology/EULAR Classification Criteria for Takayasu Arteritis. Arthritis Rheumatol 2022;74(12):1872–80.
4. Ponte C, Grayson PC, Robson JC, et al. American College of Rheumatology/EULAR Classification Criteria for Giant Cell Arteritis. Arthritis Rheumatol 2022;74(12):1881–9.
5. Robson JC, Grayson PC, Ponte C, et al. American College of Rheumatology/European Alliance of Associations for Rheumatology Classification Criteria for Granulomatosis With Polyangiitis. Arthritis Rheumatol 2022;74(3):393–9.
6. Suppiah R, Robson JC, Grayson PC, et al. American College of Rheumatology/European Alliance of Associations for Rheumatology Classification Criteria for Microscopic Polyangiitis. Arthritis Rheumatol 2022;74(3):400–6.
7. Lally L, Spiera RF. Pulmonary vasculitis. Rheum Dis Clin North Am 2015;41(2):315–31.
8. Castañer E, Alguersuari A, Andreu M, et al. Imaging findings in pulmonary vasculitis. Semin Ultrasound CT MR 2012;33(6):567–79.
9. Agarwal R, Aggarwal AN, Gupta D. Another cause of reverse halo sign: Wegener's granulomatosis. Br J Radiol 2007;80(958):849–50.
10. Ananthakrishnan L, Sharma N, Kanne JP. Wegener's granulomatosis in the chest: high-resolution CT findings. AJR Am J Roentgenol 2009;192(3):676–82.
11. Martinez Del Pero M, Sivasothy P. Vasculitis of the upper and lower airway. Best Pract Res Clin Rheumatol 2009;23(3):403–17.
12. Niles JL, Böttinger EP, Saurina GR, et al. The syndrome of lung hemorrhage and nephritis is usually an ANCA-associated condition. Arch Intern Med 1996;156(4):440–5.
13. Finkielman JD, Lee AS, Hummel AM, et al. ANCA are detectable in nearly all patients with active severe Wegener's granulomatosis. Am J Med 2007;120(7). 643.e9-14.
14. Guillevin L, Durand-Gasselin B, Cevallos R, et al. Microscopic polyangiitis: clinical and laboratory

14. findings in eighty-five patients. Arthritis Rheum 1999;42(3):421–30.
15. Sinico RA, Di Toma L, Maggiore U, et al. Prevalence and clinical significance of antineutrophil cytoplasmic antibodies in Churg-Strauss syndrome. Arthritis Rheum 2005;52(9):2926–35.
16. Falk RJ, Gross WL, Guillevin L, et al. Granulomatosis with polyangiitis (Wegener's): an alternative name for Wegener's granulomatosis. Arthritis Rheum 2011; 63(4):863–4.
17. Hellmich B, Lamprecht P, Spearpoint P, et al. New insights into the epidemiology of ANCA-associated vasculitides in Germany: results from a claims data study. Rheumatology 2021;60(10):4868–73.
18. Mohammad AJ. An update on the epidemiology of ANCA-associated vasculitis. Rheumatology 2020; 59(Supplement_3):iii42–50.
19. Seo P, Stone JH. The antineutrophil cytoplasmic antibody-associated vasculitides. Am J Med 2004; 117(1):39–50.
20. Frankel SK, Schwarz MI. The Pulmonary Vasculitides. Am J Respir Crit Care Med 2012;186(3):216–24.
21. Lally L, Spiera R. Current landscape of antineutrophil cytoplasmic antibody-associated vasculitis: classification, diagnosis, and treatment. Rheum Dis Clin N Am 2015;41(1):1–19, vii.
22. Chung MP, Yi CA, Lee HY, et al. Imaging of pulmonary vasculitis. Radiology 2010;255(2):322–41.
23. Paroli M, Gioia C, Accapezzato D. New Insights into Pathogenesis and Treatment of ANCA-Associated Vasculitis: Autoantibodies and Beyond. Antibodies 2023;12(1).
24. Lee KS, Kim TS, Fujimoto K, et al. Thoracic manifestation of Wegener's granulomatosis: CT findings in 30 patients. Eur Radiol 2003;13(1):43–51.
25. Mahmoud S, Ghosh S, Farver C, et al. Pulmonary Vasculitis: Spectrum of Imaging Appearances. Radiol Clin North Am 2016;54(6):1097–118.
26. Quinn KA, Gelbard A, Sibley C, et al. Subglottic stenosis and endobronchial disease in granulomatosis with polyangiitis. Rheumatology 2019;58(12):2203–11.
27. Martinez F, Chung JH, Digumarthy SR, et al. Common and uncommon manifestations of Wegener granulomatosis at chest CT: radiologic-pathologic correlation. Radiographics 2012;32(1):51–69.
28. Gioffredi A, Maritati F, Oliva E, et al. Eosinophilic granulomatosis with polyangiitis: an overview. Front Immunol 2014;5:549.
29. Keogh KA, Specks U. Churg-Strauss syndrome: clinical presentation, antineutrophil cytoplasmic antibodies, and leukotriene receptor antagonists. Am J Med 2003;115(4):284–90.
30. Sinico RA, Di Toma L, Maggiore U, et al. Renal involvement in Churg-Strauss syndrome. Am J Kidney Dis 2006;47(5):770–9.
31. Emmi G, Bettiol A, Gelain E, et al. Evidence-Based Guideline for the diagnosis and management of eosinophilic granulomatosis with polyangiitis. Nat Rev Rheumatol 2023;19(6):378–93.
32. Kim YK, Lee KS, Chung MP, et al. Pulmonary involvement in Churg-Strauss syndrome: an analysis of CT, clinical, and pathologic findings. Eur Radiol 2007;17(12):3157–65.
33. Neumann T, Manger B, Schmid M, et al. Cardiac involvement in Churg-Strauss syndrome: impact of endomyocarditis. Medicine (Baltim) 2009;88(4):236–43.
34. Takayasu M. A case with curious change in the central retinal vessel. Nippon Ganka Gakkai Zasshi 1908;12:554–5.
35. Matsunaga N, Hayashi K, Sakamoto I, et al. Takayasu arteritis: protean radiologic manifestations and diagnosis. Radiographics 1997;17(3):579–94.
36. Maz M, Chung SA, Abril A, et al. American College of Rheumatology/Vasculitis Foundation Guideline for the Management of Giant Cell Arteritis and Takayasu Arteritis. Arthritis Rheumatol 2021;73(8):1349–65.
37. Dejaco C, Ramiro S, Duftner C, et al. EULAR recommendations for the use of imaging in large vessel vasculitis in clinical practice. Ann Rheum Dis 2018; 77(5):636–43.
38. Ceylan N, Bayraktaroglu S, Erturk SM, et al. Pulmonary and Vascular Manifestations of Behçet Disease: Imaging Findings. Am J Roentgenol 2010;194(2): W158–64.
39. Erkan F, Gül A, Tasali E. Pulmonary manifestations of Behçet's disease. Thorax 2001;56(7):572–8.
40. Numan F, Islak C, Berkmen T, et al. Behçet disease: pulmonary arterial involvement in 15 cases. Radiology 1994;192(2):465–8.
41. Starekova J, Pirasteh A, Reeder SB. Update on gadolinium based contrast agent safety, from the AJR special series on contrast media. AJR Am J Roentgenol 2023. https://doi.org/10.2214/ajr.23.30036.
42. Manapragada PP, Andrikopoulou E, Bajaj N, et al. PET Cardiac Imaging (Perfusion, Viability, Sarcoidosis, and Infection). Radiol Clin North Am 2021;59(5): 835–52.

Congenital Pulmonary Vascular Anomalies and Disease

Alexander Phan, MD[a,*], Larry A. Latson Jr, MD, MS[a], Daniel Vargas, MD[b], Joanna G. Escalon, MD[a]

KEYWORDS

- Congenital • Pulmonary artery • Conotruncal • Pulmonary veins • Vascular anomalies • Review

KEY POINTS

- Congenital pulmonary vascular anomalies and diseases encompass a wide range of entities involving the pulmonic valve, pulmonary arteries, and/or pulmonary veins, many of which occur in the setting of additional congenital anomalies.
- Given the advancements in treatments, these patients have longer life expectancies, and therefore familiarity with these entities, including pre-operative and post-operative imaging and possible post-repair complications are imperative.
- Some entities are asymptomatic or variable in their presentation/onset and therefore radiologists may be the first to discover.
- Contrast-enhanced cross-sectional imaging, whether with computed tomography angiography or magnetic resonance angiography, should be considered the first-line modality in these adult patients and is generally sufficient to make the diagnosis, problem-solve, and perform follow-up evaluation.

INTRODUCTION

Congenital pulmonary vascular anomalies and diseases encompass a wide range of entities. This article will focus on those that are most likely encountered in adulthood, highlighting key imaging features and relevant clinical considerations. Although many occur in the setting of concurrent cardiac anomalies, the authors' discussion will be focused on the manifestations in the pulmonary arteries and veins. A list of entities discussed is outlined in **Box 1**.

PULMONARY ARTERIAL ANOMALIES
Conotruncal Anomalies

The following section will focus on the relevant findings pertaining to the pulmonic valve, main pulmonary artery (MPA), and branch pulmonary arteries in select congenital heart diseases (CHD).

Tetralogy of Fallot

Tetralogy of Fallot (TOF) is the most common cyanotic congenital disorder accounting for 7% to 10% of all CHD.[1] Anterior malposition of the

---

[a] Division of Cardiothoracic Imaging, Department of Radiology, New York-Presbyterian Hospital, Weill Cornell Medical Center, 525 East 68th Street, New York, NY 10065, USA; [b] Division of Cardiopulmonary Imaging, Department of Radiology, University of Colorado School of Medicine, 12401 East 17th Avenue, Aurora, CO 80045, USA
* Corresponding author. 525 East 68th Street, New York, NY 10065.
E-mail address: alp9138@med.cornell.edu
Twitter: @DanielVargasMD (D.V.); @JoannaEscalonMD (J.G.E.)

> **Box 1**
> **Outline of congenital pulmonary arterial and venous anomalies**
>
> Pulmonary Arterial Anomalies
>
> Conotruncal Anomalies
> - Tetralogy of Fallot
> - Pulmonary atresia
>   - Pulmonary atresia with ventricular septal defect
>   - Pulmonary atresia with intact ventricular septum
> - Truncus arteriosus
>
> Other Pulmonary Arterial Anomalies
> - Patent ductus arteriosus
> - Pulmonary artery stenosis
>   - Valvular stenosis
>   - Subvalvular stenosis
>   - Supravalvular stenosis
> - Pulmonary sling
> - Proximal interruption of the pulmonary artery
> - Crisscross or crossed pulmonary arteries
> - Pulmonary arteriovenous malformation
>
> Pulmonary Venous Anomalies
> - Normal variants
> - Total anomalous pulmonary venous return
> - Partial anomalous pulmonary venous return
>   - Scimitar syndrome
> - Levoatriocardinal vein
> - Meandering pulmonary vein
> - Varix

conal septum gives rise to the 4 classic features: right ventricular outflow tract (RVOT)/pulmonary artery (PA) obstruction, overriding aorta, outlet/membranous ventricular septal defect (VSD), and consequent right ventricular (RV) hypertrophy.[2,3] The severity and onset are mainly determined by the degree of RVOT/pulmonary artery obstruction, which can range from mild RVOT obstruction (with or without pulmonic valvular stenosis) to pulmonary atresia.[2] When there is severe pulmonary stenosis or atresia, pulmonic blood flow may be dependent on a patent ductus arteriosus (PDA) or major aortopulmonary collateral arteries (MAPCAs). The location of the pulmonary outflow tract stenoses/obstruction is variable and can affect the branch pulmonary arteries (Fig. 1A–C).[2]

Corrective surgery involves VSD closure and relieving the RVOT/pulmonary obstruction. Typically, a transannular patch made of autologous pericardium, Dacron, or Gore-Tex is used to augment and increase the diameter of the RVOT (see Fig. 1). The patch can also be extended to the main and/or branch pulmonary arteries to increase their diameter.[1]

Computed tomography (CT) and MRI are both helpful in the pre-operative and post-operative assessment. Post-operative imaging can reveal VSD patch leaks, RVOT obstruction, residual/recurrent branch pulmonary artery stenosis, and aortopulmonary collaterals. Approximately 50% of repaired TOF will undergo reoperation within 30 years for pulmonary valve replacement due to valvular dysfunction, most commonly pulmonary regurgitation.[1]

Pulmonary atresia
Pulmonary atresia is a lack of communication between the RV and the pulmonary arteries either due to muscular atresia (overgrowth of the infundibulum and RV apex) or from valvular atresia.[4] It can be divided into those with a ventricular septal defect (PA-VSD) and those with an intact ventricular septum (PA-IVS).

Pulmonary atresia with ventricular septal defect
In pulmonary atresia with ventricular septal defect (PA-VSD), often considered a severe form of TOF, the main and branch pulmonary arteries are often atretic or hypoplastic and may be discontinuous with one another (Fig. 2A–E). This necessitates the need for extracardiac sources of pulmonary blood flow, usually a PDA or MAPCAs.[4] PA-VSD can be classified into 3 types based on the source of pulmonary blood supply:[5]

1. Type A with blood supply from the native pulmonary artery
2. Type B with blood supply from both native pulmonary artery and MAPCAs
3. Type C with MAPCAs only

MAPCAs are large arterial collateral vessels which typically arise from the descending thoracic aorta but can also arise from the aortic arch and arch vessels, abdominal aorta, or more rarely, from other systemic arteries such as the coronary arteries.[1] MAPCAs then anastomose with the pulmonary arteries in the mediastinum and hila at the lobar or subsegmental level to provide blood flow into the lungs (see Fig. 2).[1,4] PDA and MAPCAs will typically not supply the same side of the lung.[4] PDA can supply one or both branch pulmonary arteries.

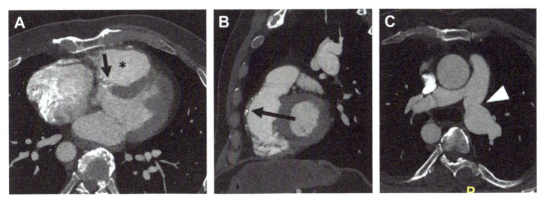

Fig. 1. Tetralogy of Fallot (TOF). A 56-year-old male with TOF repaired at age 8. (*A-C*) Contrast-enhanced computed tomography (CT) shows right aortic arch, dilated right ventricle (RV) (*A, asterisk*), partially calcified ventricular septal defect (VSD) and right ventricular outflow tract (RVOT) patches (*A, B, arrows*) with unobstructed RVOT, absence of pulmonary valve leaflet tissue, and mild narrowing of the proximal left pulmonary artery (PA) (*C, arrowhead*) with post-stenotic dilation.

Management can be broadly divided into rehabilitation, unifocalization, or a combination of both. Rehabilitation is aimed at creating a shunt to promote growth of the native pulmonary arteries allowing later definitive repair with an extracardiac RV-to-PA conduit.[2,5] Unifocalization is aimed at ligating, mobilizing, and anastomosing the ipsilateral MAPCAs to each other and incorporating them into the native pulmonary artery.[5]

CT or MRI is the key for delineating the pulmonary arterial anatomy to direct the repair approach. The following should be reported:[4]

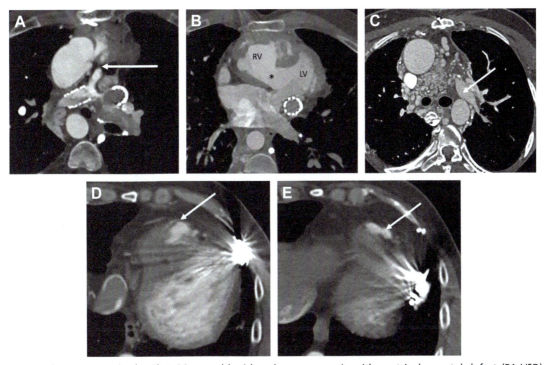

Fig. 2. Pulmonary atresia. (*A, B*) A 26-year-old with pulmonary atresia with ventricular septal defect (PA-VSD) showing atretic main pulmonary artery (MPA) not connecting to the RV (*arrow*) and large VSD (*asterisk*). (*C*) A 32-year-old with pulmonary atresia with intact ventricular septum (PA-IVS) demonstrating discontinuous branch pulmonary arteries (*arrow* on the left pulmonary artery [LPA]) and numerous major aortopulmonary collateral arteries (MAPCAs). (*D, E*) Patient with PA-IVS and coronary sinusoid communicating with the RV (*arrows*).

- Level at which the atresia occurs
- Degree of the hypoplasia
- Connections between the MPA and the branch arteries
- Number, size, origin, and course of MAPCAs
- Extracardiac sources of blood flow

In the post-operative assessment, special attention should be made to the main and branch pulmonary arteries (for stenoses) and MAPCAs (for stenoses, aneurysm, or associated pulmonary hemorrhage).[6]

Pulmonary atresia with intact ventricular septum

In the absence of a VSD, PA-IVS requires an alternative blood flow route to the pulmonic circulation—generally via a patent foramen ovale (PFO) or atrial septal defect (ASD) and then to pulmonary arteries via a PDA. Patients are therefore PDA dependent and present earlier with cyanosis in the first 48 hours of life as the ductus arteriosus closes.[4] In contradistinction to PA-VSD, the RV is often hypoplastic and small as the absence of shunting inhibits RV cavity growth.

PA-IVS is associated with coronary artery anomalies, including ventriculocoronary sinusoids/fistulae and coronary stenosis/atresia. Ventriculocoronary sinusoids/fistulae are intramyocardial channels that directly connect the coronary artery to the ventricular cavity while bypassing a capillary bed (see **Fig. 2**). As a result, the coronary system becomes RV flow dependent and elevated RV flows must be maintained to provide adequate coronary perfusion, which can affect the surgical approach for repair.[4]

Truncus arteriosus

Truncus arterious (TA) is an overriding common arterial trunk with a single semilunar valve that gives rise to both the aorta and at least 1 pulmonary artery thus supplying the systemic, pulmonic, and coronary circulation.[2,3] There are multiple variations depending on the origins and branching pattern of the pulmonary arteries. For example, the MPA can arise from the common trunk, branch pulmonary arteries can be discontinuous and arise directly from the common trunk with separate ostia, or one branch can arise from the trunk while the other is supplied by a PDA or MAPCAs. TA can be associated with a host of cardiovascular anomalies including VSD, interrupted arch, and anomalous pulmonary venous return, as well as genetic syndromes, most commonly DiGeorge syndrome.[2]

TA is diagnosed in the neonatal period and typically surgically corrected within the first few weeks of life. Corrective surgery involves separating the pulmonary artery from the common trunk and reconnecting it to the RV via a conduit, realigning the common trunk with the left ventricle (LV) to create a neo-aorta, and patch closure of the VSD. Branch pulmonary arteries and MAPCAs can be mobilized and joined to the pulmonary artery/conduit if needed (**Fig. 3**A, B). CT or MRI is valuable in the post-operative period to evaluate for neo-aortic valve stenosis or regurgitation, RV-to-PA conduit stenosis, and VSD leak.[1]

Other Pulmonary Arterial Anomalies

Patent ductus arteriosus

The ductus arteriosus is a short vessel that connects the proximal descending aorta (at the isthmus) to the MPA during fetal development.[4,7] In utero, it delivers deoxygenated blood from the MPA to the thoracic aorta. After birth, the ductus arteriosus involutes, forming the ligamentum

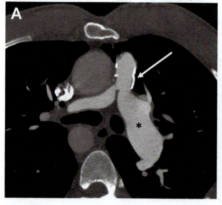
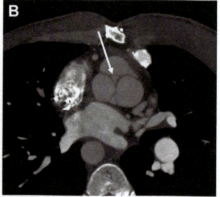

Fig. 3. Truncus arteriosus. A 29-year-old with repaired truncus arteriosus with (*A*) calcified right ventricle-to-pulmonary artery conduit (*arrow*), distal MPA and branch pulmonary artery stenoses, and post-stenotic dilation left PA (*asterisk*) as well as (*B*) non-coapting (*arrow*) thickened truncal valve leaflets with aortic root aneurysm and severe aortic regurgitation.

arteriosum. If the ductus persists more than 48 hours after birth, it is considered a PDA. Most cases are sporadic, although PDAs are associated with prematurity, viral infections such as rubella, and CHD. In ductal-dependent CHD, the ductus can be maintained open using prostaglandins.[7]

Most small PDAs are asymptomatic and incidentally found (**Fig. 4**A–D). Moderate PDAs can become symptomatic after developing hypertension in adulthood, as the increased left-to-right shunt can lead to symptoms of heart failure. Large PDAs present in infancy to early childhood with congestive heart failure (see **Fig. 4**). If unrepaired, they can develop severe pulmonary hypertension and Eisenmenger syndrome with reversal of the flow to a right-to-left shunt.[7]

Echocardiography is the mainstay for diagnosis in infants and children. Radiographs are typically normal in those with smaller PDAs, while larger PDAs lead to enlargement of the MPA and left-sided chambers due to over-circulation. Contrast-enhanced CT and MRI allow assessment of the PDA configuration by the Krichenko classification, useful for pre-closure planning. Phase-contrast imaging on MRI allows shunt volume and fraction quantification.[7,8] Potential pitfalls include a calcified ligamentum arteriosum (confirmed on non-contrast CT) and a ductus diverticulum (focal bulge at the level of the isthmus without connection to the MPA).[7]

Silent or hemodynamically insignificant PDAs may not warrant any treatment. Medical management is favored in neonates. Some require surgical ligation or transcatheter closure.[9] Surgical ligation is the primary option for premature infants or those with exceptionally large PDA and unsuitable anatomy for transcatheter closure.[7]

Pulmonary artery stenosis

Pulmonary artery stenosis is categorized into either valvular, subvalvular, or supravalvular, in order of frequency. Most (95%) are congenital.[4,10]

Valvular stenosis In valvular stenosis, the pulmonic leaflets are thickened or partially fused, resulting in luminal narrowing and increased flow velocities and pressure gradients across the valve. On radiography (**Fig. 5**A–C), CT, and MRI, there will be asymmetric enlargement of the MPA and left pulmonary artery (LPA) due to an eccentric flow jet toward the LPA leading to post-stenotic dilation (see **Fig. 5**). The right pulmonary artery (RPA) will be normal in caliber. ECG-gated CT or MRI allows assessment of valve morphology, and MRI allows evaluation of RV function/morphology and flow quantification across the valve with phase contrast imaging.[4]

Treatments include balloon valvuloplasty and pulmonic valve replacement (via open surgical or trans-catheter approach).[4]

Subvalvular stenosis Subvalvular stenosis usually occurs due to diffuse thickening of the infundibulum/conus arteriosus. Less common causes include anomalous muscle band, moderator

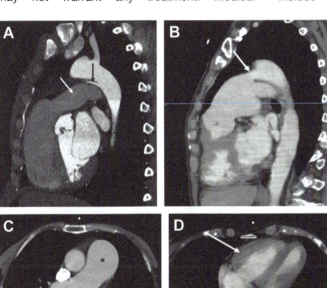

Fig. 4. Patent ductus arteriosus (PDA). (A) A 20-year-old with small patent ductus arteriosus (black arrow) and jet of contrast in the MPA (white arrow). (B–D) A 60-year-old with unrepaired PDA (B, arrow) and Eisenmenger syndrome with resultant MPA dilation (C, asterisk) and RV hypertrophy (D, arrow).

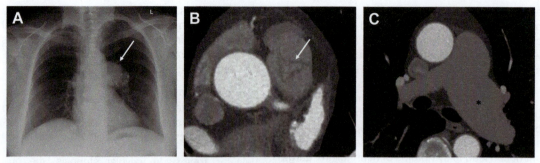

Fig. 5. Congenital pulmonary valve stenosis. (*A*) A 72-year-old with asymmetrically enlarged main and left PA (*arrow*). (*B, C*) A 64-year-old with mildly thickened pulmonic valve leaflets (*B, arrow*) and enlarged main and left PA (*C, asterisk*).

band hypertrophy, and idiopathic RV hypertrophy. Subvalvular stenosis usually occurs in the setting of other CHD, most commonly TOF.[11]

Supravalvular stenosis In supravalvular stenosis, the MPA or branch pulmonary arteries are abnormally narrowed with or without post-stenotic dilation. Depending on the severity, it can lead to RV hypertrophy, dysfunction, and eventually failure (**Fig. 6**A–D). Supravalvular stenosis is commonly seen with other CHD as well as Williams, Alagille, Ehlers-Danlos, and post-rubella syndromes. Treatment is primarily angioplasty with or without stenting (see **Fig. 6**A–D).[4]

Pulmonary sling
Left pulmonary artery sling occurs when the LPA arises from the posterior aspect of the RPA and then courses between the distal trachea and

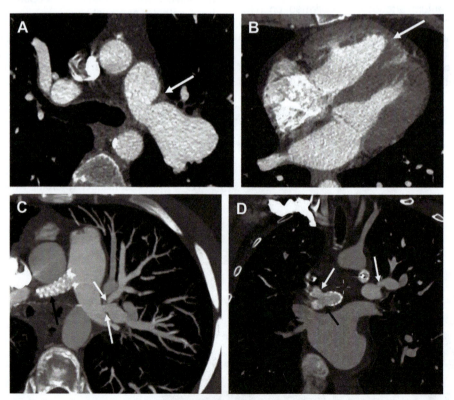

Fig. 6. Supravalvular pulmonary artery stenosis. (*A, B*) A 44-year-old with congenital rubella and pulmonic stenosis demonstrating LPA stenosis (*A, arrow*) with post-stenotic dilation and RV hypertrophy (*B, arrow*). (*C, D*) A 24-year-old with Keutel syndrome and multiple central and peripheral pulmonary artery stenoses (*white arrows*) and central right pulmonary artery (RPA) stent (*black arrows*).

esophagus to reach the left hilum.[4] Pulmonary slings are classified into 2 types.

- Type I: Sling occurs above the carina (T4-5 level) and the airway caliber is normal but the distal trachea and right main bronchus may be compressed by the sling (Fig. 7A, B).
- Type II: Sling occurs more inferior (T5-6 level) and is associated with a T-shaped pseudocarina and right bridging bronchus arising from the left. It is also associated with long-segment airway stenosis with complete cartilaginous rings (the "ring-sling complex"), unilateral or bilateral pulmonary overinflation, and hypoplastic or absent right lung.[12] Type II has higher morbidity and mortality, often presenting in the first weeks of life with severe obstructive airway symptoms.[4]

On radiographs, the sling may mimic a mediastinal mass on the frontal view. On the lateral view, a rounded opacity occurs between the trachea and esophagus (Fig. 7C, D).[10] On esophagraphy, a sling is the only condition causing anterior indentation on the esophagus as it courses between the trachea and the esophagus. Asymmetric hyperinflation of the right lung with or without tracheal narrowing may also occur. CT and MRI can confirm the diagnosis and allow evaluation of the tracheobronchial branching pattern, presence of complete cartilaginous rings (rounded configuration of the airways), and the presence and length of stenoses. Repair involves reimplantation of the LPA to the MPA and repair of any concomitant tracheobronchial stenoses or rings.[3,4,12]

Proximal interruption of the pulmonary artery

Proximal interruption of the pulmonary artery (PIPA) is when either the right or left pulmonary artery abruptly ends in the mediastinum before supplying the lung. The term *interruption* is favored over *absence* or *atresia* given that the intrapulmonary arteries are maintained.[4,13]

The affected side is typically opposite the aortic arch. Right PIPA with left aortic arch is more common and typically isolated. Left PIPA with right aortic arch is usually associated with other anomalies. Intrapulmonary arteries are supplied through systemic collateral vessels, including bronchial arteries/MAPCAs and transpleurally from intercostal, internal mammary, subclavian, and brachiocephalic arteries.[4,13]

On radiographs, the affected hemithorax will have volume loss (Fig. 8A). On CT, the affected pulmonary artery will be absent or terminate within 1 cm of its origin. The bronchial arteries and systemic collaterals are hypertrophic. Transpleural collaterals result in serrated pleural thickening and subpleural parenchymal bands (Fig. 8B). Acquired

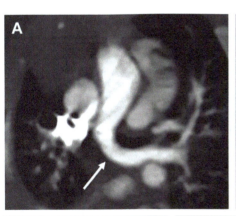
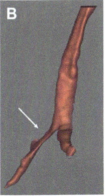
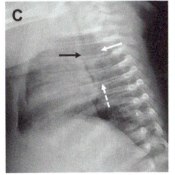
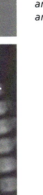

Fig. 7. Pulmonary sling (pre-surgical). (A, B) A 14-day-old female with computed tomography (CT) showing pulmonary sling (A, arrow) and 3-D reconstructions with narrowing/flattening of the proximal left mainstem bronchus (B, arrow). (C, D) A 1-month 20-day-old female with pulmonary sling with chest radiograph (C) and CT (D) showing an ovoid opacity (*dashed arrow*) corresponding to the pulmonary sling between the trachea (*black arrow*) and the esophagus (*white arrow*).

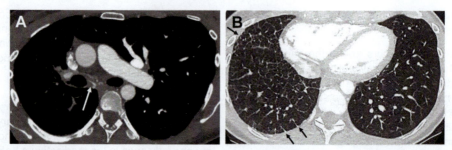

Fig. 8. Proximal interruption of the pulmonary artery (PIPA). Right PIPA with contrast-enhanced CT showing (A) completely atretic right MPA and multiple bronchial artery collaterals (*arrow*) and (B) small right lung with thickened, serrated pleura, and interlobular septal thickening (*arrows*) due to transpleural collaterals.

causes of proximal pulmonary artery obstruction should be excluded, including chronic pulmonary thromboembolism, vasculitis, and fibrosing mediastinitis. Scimitar and Swyer-James-McLeod syndromes can have similar appearances on radiographs, but CT will differentiate.[13]

Patients may present with recurrent pulmonary infections, hemorrhage, and dyspnea. Hemoptysis is reported in 10% to 20% cases due to rupture of hypertrophied collateral vessels. Prognosis is determined by the degree of pulmonary hypertension, which affects 19% to 25% of cases.[4,13]

Crisscross or crossed pulmonary arteries

Crossed pulmonary arteries (CPA) is an uncommon anatomic variant, the exact prevalence of which is unknown given only a few hospital-based studies.[14] CPA is usually associated with other congenital anomalies, including VSD, TOF, TA, right aortic arch, and DiGeorge syndrome.[15]

In CPA, the ostium of the LPA lies to the right and is superior to the ostium of the RPA resulting in the proximal arteries crossing as they course to their respective lungs (**Fig. 9**A–C). Care should also be taken to not mistaken CPA for a pulmonary sling.

As it has no functional consequences, its main significance is for surgical planning, as the altered anatomy may create difficulties for certain procedures.[15]

Pulmonary arteriovenous malformation

Pulmonary arteriovenous malformations (PAVMs) are abnormal direct connections between a pulmonary artery and a pulmonary vein bypassing the capillary bed, thus resulting in a right-to-left shunt. A total of 80% to 90% of PAVMs are associated with hereditary hemorrhagic telangiectasia, an autosomal dominant disorder leading to AVMs in multiple organs.[16] PAVMs can also occur in hepatopulmonary syndrome due to chronic liver disease and in CHD after cavopulmonary shunt (ie, Fontan) procedures, potentially due to a lack or imbalanced distribution of hepatic venous flow to the pulmonary arteries (the "hepatic factor" hypothesis).[17]

PAVMs may be radiographically occult or appear as a nodular opacity. Pulmonary arterial phase CT is the preferred modality to identify PAVMs and evaluate their location, number, size, and morphology. Use of maximum intensity projections (MIPs) is especially helpful in highlighting the vascular connections (**Fig. 10**). Special note

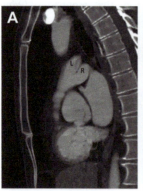 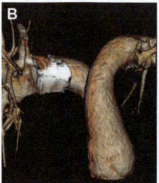 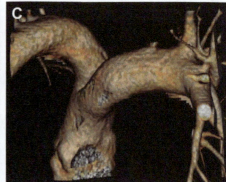

Fig. 9. Crossed pulmonary arteries. A 50-year-old male with Loeys-Dietz syndrome and (A) sagittal CT showing the left PA (*L*) directly above the right PA (*R*) with anterior (B) and posterior (C) 3-D reconstructions.

Congenital Pulmonary Vascular Anomalies and Disease

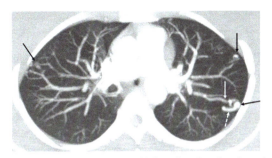

Fig. 10. PAVM. A 26-year-old female who developed shortness of breath after normal spontaneous vaginal delivery. CT showed multiple pulmonary arteriovenous malformations with niduses (*black arrows*), arterial feeder (*white arrow*), and draining vein (*dashed arrow*).

should be made to describe the caliber size and number of feeding arteries.[16]

Simple PAVMs consist of 1 or more feeding pulmonary arteries from a *single* segmental pulmonary artery. Small PAVMs can initially present as groundglass opacities with small discrete vessels that eventually progress and grow to true PAVMs. Complex PAVMs are supplied by *multiple* segmental pulmonary arteries. PAVMs can also be referred to as "diffuse" when they have *numerous* small feeding arteries with or without more discrete simple and complex PAVMs.[16,18]

PAVMs can result in paradoxic embolization leading to stroke, transient ischemic attack, systemic embolism, or brain abscess. PAVMs lack normal elasticity in the vessel walls, which can lead to hemothorax and hemoptysis, of particular concern in pregnant woman (reported 1% risk of maternal mortality). Standard treatment is transcatheter embolization utilizing an array of coils and plugs. Historically, PAVMs were treated if the feeding pulmonary artery diameter was at least 3 mm. However, given that small PAVMs can still develop complications and many grow, the consensus now is to treat most PAVMs if they can be successfully catheterized.[16]

PULMONARY VENOUS ANOMALIES
Normal Variants

Pulmonary venous anatomy is highly variable regarding number of veins and ostial arrangement and therefore should be discussed in terms of commonality rather than what is "normal." The most common pattern (57%–82%) is 4 pulmonary vein ostia–right and left superior pulmonary veins (draining the upper and middle lobes/lingula) and inferior pulmonary veins (draining the lower lobes). The most common variants include common ostium and supernumerary pulmonary veins, which result from under-incorporation or over-incorporation of the veins during embryologic development.[19]

A common ostium is when the superior and inferior veins converge to share a single ostium and is most common on the left.

A supernumerary pulmonary vein is any vein seen in addition to the 4 standard veins. A separate right middle vein is seen in 9% to 27% of people. A "right top vein" is a small vein passing posterior and medial to the bronchus intermedius or right main bronchus before inserting into the left atrium (LA), usually draining the right upper lobe posterior segment or right lower lobe superior segment (**Fig. 11**A, B). Mention of pulmonary venous variants is important in pre-operative planning for catheter-ablation procedures as they may be sources of atrial fibrillation.[19]

Total Anomalous Pulmonary Venous Return

In total anomalous pulmonary venous return (TAPVR), all pulmonary veins drain into the systemic venous circulation instead of their normal drainage into the LA. TAPVR is classified into types based on the anatomic level of their drainage, as listed in order of frequency:[20,21]

- Supracardiac: Pulmonary veins first drain into a confluence posterior to the LA before ascending superiorly via an anomalous

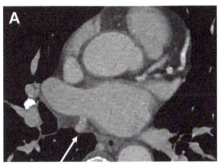
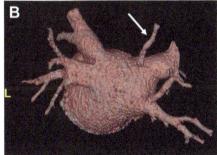

Fig. 11. Right top vein (*arrow*) on (*A*) contrast-enhanced CT and (*B*) 3-D reconstructions, a normal anatomic variant.

vertical vein which drains into the left brachiocephalic vein (Fig. 12A–C).
- Cardiac: Pulmonary veins drain directly into the posterior wall of the right atrium (RA) or via the coronary sinus.
- Infracardiac: Pulmonary veins drain below the diaphragm via a descending vein to either the portal venous system (most common) or systemic veins (inferior vena cava [IVC], hepatic vein, or azygos system) (Fig. 13A, B).
- Mixed: Pulmonary veins drain to 2 or more different locations.

Pulmonary venous obstruction can occur with all types and is important to recognize as it can influence the timing of and approach to surgical repair. Obstruction occurs most frequently in the infracardiac type (up to 78% of patients), usually at the level of the diaphragm.[20]

On radiographs, the "snowman" or "figure of 8" appearance occurs with the supracardiac type due to mediastinal widening from the dilated left brachiocephalic vein and superior vena cava (SVC) (see Fig. 12).[22] Contrast-enhanced CT or MR allows confirmation, pre-procedural planning, and evaluation of associated anomalies.[20]

Partial Anomalous Pulmonary Venous Return

Partial anomalous pulmonary venous return (PAPVR) occurs when at least 1 but *not all* pulmonary veins drain into the systemic venous circulation. Like TAPVR, it can be classified based on the anatomic level of drainage (supracardiac, cardiac, infracardiac) with cardiac type being the most common. Right upper lobe (RUL) PAPVR is most common, usually draining into the right atrium or SVC, or less commonly into the coronary sinus, azygos, or IVC.[20] RUL PAPVR is highly associated (80%–90%) with an SVC-type sinus venosus ASD and care must be taken to search for both anomalies when either one is identified (Fig. 14A–C).[20,23]

Left PAPVR usually drains into the left brachiocephalic vein via a vertical vein, less commonly into the coronary sinus or hemiazygos system. The vertical vein occupies the left para-aortic or prevascular region where typically only mediastinal fat is present. The differential diagnosis for any vessel in this region is PAPVR versus persistent left SVC, distinguished by following the course of the vessel.[20]

PAPVR results in a low-pressure left-to-right shunt, similar to an ASD, but many patients are asymptomatic. If unrepaired, PAPVR causes chronic volume load on the right heart, which can lead to RV dilation and failure. Development and severity of symptoms depends on the size of the anomalous vein (how much lung it drains) and degree of shunting. Qp/Qs greater than 1.5:1 generally prompts surgical repair by direct reimplantation or interatrial baffling. Transcatheter endovascular techniques have also been employed.[23]

Scimitar syndrome

Also called "hypogenetic lung syndrome or congenital venolobar syndrome," scimitar syndrome is a subset of right PAPVR that involves venous drainage of part or all of the right lung into the supra-diaphragmatic or infra-diaphragmatic IVC (most common), however, occasionally into the hepatic veins, azygos system, portal vein, right atrium or coronary sinus (Fig. 15).[21] On radiographs, this anomalous connection results in the characteristic curved linear opacity lateral to the right cardiac border known as the *scimitar sign*.[20] The complete constellation of this syndrome also includes right lung hypoplasia, dextrocardia, RPA hypoplasia, and anomalous systemic arterial supply to the right lower lobe. The term "*scimitar variant*" has been used to describe those that do not meet all these

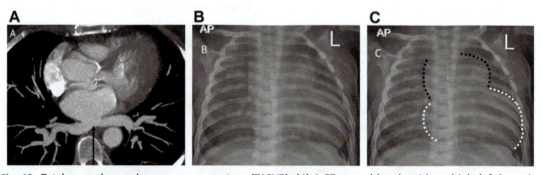

Fig. 12. Total anomalous pulmonary venous return (TAPVR). (*A*) A 57-year-old male with multiple left heart lesions, including "forme fruste" TAPVR (unobstructed) (*arrow*), bicuspid aortic valve, prior coarctation repair (not pictured). (*B, C*) A 2-month-15-day-old male with supracardiac TAPVR; dilated superior vena cava (SVC) and left brachiocephalic vein resulting in the "snowman" or "Figure of 8" appearance on CXR.

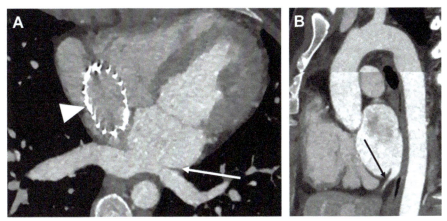

Fig. 13. TAPVR. A 36-year-old with infradiaphragmatic TAPVR repaired in infancy. CT shows repaired TAPVR (opening of common confluence of pulmonary veins into the left atrium), mild residual narrowing of the common left pulmonary vein (A, arrow), partially imaged stent IVC to right atrium (A, arrowhead), and remnant of the infradiaphragmatic TAPVR coursing from below diaphragm up into the left atrium (B, arrow).

typical features.[24] Additional lesser associations include accessory diaphragms, diaphragmatic hernias, bronchial anomalies, pulmonary lobation anomalies, "horseshoe" lung, hemivertebrae, and genitourinary tract anomalies.[20–22]

Levoatriocardinal vein

Levoatriocardinal vein is an anomalous connection formed between the LA or pulmonary vein to a systemic vein. It is derived from failed regression of the embryologic cardinal veins. It typically occurs in the setting of left heart obstructive lesions, such as hypoplastic left heart or mitral stenosis/atresia and is believed to function as a "pop-off channel" for the LA by allowing a decompressive pathway for pulmonary venous blood. Rarely, an isolated levoatriocardinal vein can be seen in an otherwise normal heart.[25]

Care should be taken to not mistake this entity for PAPVR. The levoatriocardinal vein connects the LA or pulmonary vein to the systemic vein. However, the key distinction is that the pulmonary vein (from which the levoatriocardinal vein can originate) maintains a normal connection the LA (Fig. 16). If there is no connection between the pulmonary vein and the LA, then it is a PAPVR. CT or MRI best allows evaluation of the origin, course, and drainage of the vein. The majority originate from the LA followed by the upper pulmonary veins with equal propensity for either side. It most commonly drains into the left brachiocephalic vein, followed by the right SVC, jugular veins, and left SVC.[25]

Levoatriocardinal veins result in a left-to-right shunt, which is typically small and does not usually require treatment. However, the shunt can be bidirectional and lead to paradoxic embolism thus prompting endovascular plugging.[25]

Meandering Pulmonary Vein

Meandering pulmonary vein (MPV) also known as "pseudo-scimitar syndrome," consists of an anomalous right pulmonary vein, which takes a

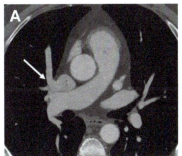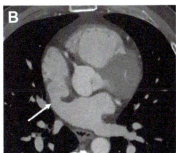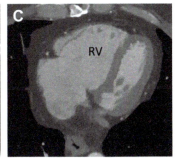

Fig. 14. Partial anomalous pulmonary venous return (PAPVR). A 57-year-old male with PAPVR with axial contrast-enhanced CT showing PAPVR (A, arrow), sinus venosus atrial septal defect (B, arrow), and dilated RV (C).

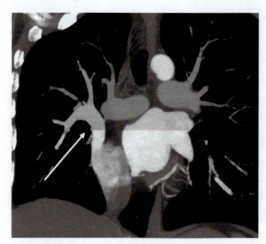

Fig. 15. Scimitar syndrome. A 53-year-old male with large anomalous vein draining the hypoplastic right lung into the supradiaphragmatic inferior vena cava (IVC) (*arrow*).

torturous course through the right lung mimicking a scimitar-shape but ultimately drains normally into the LA (**Fig. 17**). MPV can be associated with right lung hypoplasia and dextrocardia.[20,22] There are reported cases of the anomalous pulmonary vein draining into both the LA and the IVC simultaneously, which has led to confusion as whether to classify these as scimitar variant, MPV, or coexisting classic scimitar and MPV. Thus, these entities likely represent a spectrum of pulmonary venous anomalies with a common embryologic basis.[26]

On radiographs, MPV can also present with the scimitar sign; however, CT or MRI will confirm the connection to the LA.

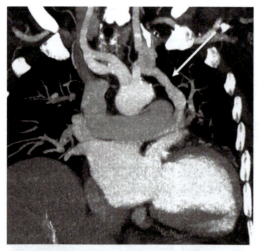

Fig. 16. Levoatriocardinal vein. A 72-year-old male with incidentally found anomalous connection (*arrow*) between the left superior pulmonary vein and left brachiocephalic vein.

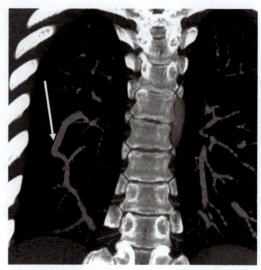

Fig. 17. Meandering vein. An 18-year-old with pulmonary sequestration (not pictured) and anomalous right pulmonary vein taking torturous course through the right lung (*arrow*) but draining normally into the left atrium.

Varix

Pulmonary venous varix is abnormal localized dilation of a pulmonary vein, most commonly at its entrance to the LA.[20,27] Incidence is unknown but considered very rare with <80 case reports as of 2011.[27] It can be congenital or acquired, most commonly occurring in the right lower lobe, followed by the left upper, right upper, right middle, and left lower lobes.[27] The morphology has been classified into confluent type (localized at the entrance of the LA, most common) (**Fig. 18**), saccular type (localized, ovoid), and tortuous type (extensive). While acquired types can be symptomatic, congenital varices are typically asymptomatic,

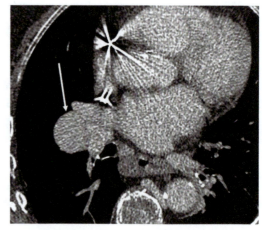

Fig. 18. Venous varix. Incidental dilation of the right superior pulmonary vein (*arrow*).

do not progress, or have complications, and do not require treatment.[28]

On radiographs, the confluent type can present as a lobulated mass or nodule adjacent to the heart.[20] CT or MRI can confirm the diagnosis. The main differential diagnosis is a PAVM, easily distinguished by the lack of a pulmonary arterial connection.[27]

SUMMARY

The aim of this article is to provide a digestible overview of a daunting and diverse topic spanning both pulmonary arterial and venous anomalies. Given advancements in treatment, patients with congenital anomalies are having longer life expectancies, and practicing radiologists are bound to come across these patients during their daily practice. Therefore, it is imperative to develop a familiarity with these entities, including pre-operative and post-operative imaging findings and possible post-repair complications. As some of these entities are asymptomatic or variable in their severity and onset, radiologists may be the first to make the diagnosis.

CLINICS CARE POINTS

- By adulthood, most patients with conotruncal anomalies will have already been diagnosed and undergone some sort of repair, therefore the radiologist's primary role is the post-operative assessment, especially any post-repair complications.
- While MAPCAs and other collaterals are often beneficial as a form of natural compensation, they also come with their own inherent risk and complications, such as aneurysms, stenoses, and hemorrhage, and should be assessed on both pre-operative and post-operative imaging.
- While some entities can be isolated findings, the majority are often associated with additional concurrent anomalies (ie, cardiac, vascular, or tracheobronchial), thus care should be taken to avoid "satisfaction of search" error.
- Some of these vascular anomalies may mimic masses or each other on radiography. Contrast-enhanced cross-sectional imaging (CTA or MRA) will reveal the correct diagnosis.
- While both CT and MRI can highlight the anatomy, MRI has the added benefit of assessing ventricular function, flow dynamics, and shunt quantification.

DISCLOSURES

The authors have nothing to disclose.

REFERENCES

1. Kumar P, Bhatia M. Role of CT in the Pre- and Postoperative Assessment of Conotruncal Anomalies. Radiol Cardiothorac Imaging 2022;4(3):e210089. Published 2022 Jun 30.
2. Newman B, Alkhori N. Congenital central pulmonary artery anomalies: Part 1. Pediatr Radiol 2020;50(8): 1022–9.
3. Zucker EJ. Cross-sectional imaging of congenital pulmonary artery anomalies. Int J Cardiovasc Imaging 2019;35(8):1535–48.
4. Escalon JG, Browne LP, Bang TJ, et al. Congenital anomalies of the pulmonary arteries: an imaging overview. Br J Radiol 2019;92(1093):20180185.
5. Soquet J, Barron DJ, d'Udekem Y. A Review of the Management of Pulmonary Atresia, Ventricular Septal Defect, and Major Aortopulmonary Collateral Arteries. Ann Thorac Surg 2019;108(2):601–12.
6. Abdel Razek AAK, Al-Marsafawy H, Elmansy M. Imaging of Pulmonary Atresia With Ventricular Septal Defect. J Comput Assist Tomogr 2019;43(6):906–11.
7. Lee SJ, Yoo SM, Son MJ, et al. The Patent Ductus Arteriosus in Adults with Special Focus on Role of CT. Diagnostics (Basel) 2021;11(12):2394. Published 2021 Dec 19.
8. Rajiah P, Kanne JP. Cardiac MRI: Part 1, cardiovascular shunts. AJR Am J Roentgenol 2011;197(4): W603–20.
9. May LA, Masand PM, Qureshi AM, et al. The ductus arteriosus: a review of embryology to intervention. Pediatr Radiol 2023;53(3):509–22.
10. Carter BW, Lichtenberger JP, Wu CC. Congenital abnormalities of the pulmonary arteries in adults. AJR Am J Roentgenol 2014;202(4):W308–13.
11. Vadher AB, Shaw M, Pandey NN, et al. Stenotic lesions of pulmonary arteries: imaging evaluation using multidetector computed tomography angiography. Clin Imaging 2021;69:17–26.
12. Newman B, Alkhori N. Congenital central pulmonary artery anomalies: Part 2. Pediatr Radiol 2020;50(8): 1030–40.
13. Castañer E, Gallardo X, Rimola J, et al. Congenital and acquired pulmonary artery anomalies in the adult: radiologic overview. Radiographics 2006; 26(2):349–71.
14. Alhassan AA, Shati AA, Al-Ahmari SM, et al. A neonate with crossed pulmonary arteries: a case report and literature review of 115 cases worldwide. Cardiol Young 2022;32(8):1196–201.
15. Mastromoro G, Calcagni G, Vignaroli W, et al. Crossed pulmonary arteries: An underestimated cardiovascular variant with a strong association with

16. Kaufman CS, McDonald J, Balch H, et al. Pulmonary Arteriovenous Malformations: What the Interventional Radiologist Should Know. Semin Intervent Radiol 2022;39(3):261–70. Published 2022 Aug 31.
17. Ohuchi H, Mori A, Nakai M, et al. Pulmonary Arteriovenous Fistulae After Fontan Operation: Incidence, Clinical Characteristics, and Impact on All-Cause Mortality. Front Pediatr 2022;10:713219. Published 2022 Jun 9.
18. Gill SS, Roddie ME, Shovlin CL, et al. Pulmonary arteriovenous malformations and their mimics. Clin Radiol 2015;70(1):96–110.
19. Hassani C, Saremi F. Comprehensive Cross-sectional Imaging of the Pulmonary Veins. Radiographics 2017;37(7):1928–54.
20. Abdel Razek AAK, Al-Marsafawy H, Elmansy M, et al. Computed Tomography Angiography and Magnetic Resonance Angiography of Congenital Anomalies of Pulmonary Veins. J Comput Assist Tomogr 2019;43(3):399–405.
21. Pandey NN, Sharma A, Jagia P. Imaging of anomalous pulmonary venous connections by multidetector CT angiography using third-generation dual source CT scanner. Br J Radiol 2018;91(1092):20180298.
22. Katre R, Burns SK, Murillo H, et al. Anomalous pulmonary venous connections. Semin Ultrasound CT MR 2012;33(6):485–99.
23. Türkvatan A, Güzeltaş A, Tola HT, et al. Multidetector Computed Tomographic Angiography Imaging of Congenital Pulmonary Venous Anomalies: A Pictorial Review. Can Assoc Radiol J 2017;68(1):66–76.
24. Bo I, Carvalho JS, Cheasty E, et al. Variants of the scimitar syndrome. Cardiol Young 2016;26(5):941–7.
25. Agarwal PP, Mahani MG, Lu JC, et al. Levoatriocardinal Vein and Mimics: Spectrum of Imaging Findings. AJR Am J Roentgenol 2015;205(2):W162–71.
26. Lee M, Jeon KN, Park MJ, et al. Meandering pulmonary veins: Two case reports. Medicine (Baltimore) 2020;99(16):e19815.
27. Yamaguchi B, Kodama Y, Watanabe K, et al. Pulmonary varix clearly demonstrated by 3D-CT before pulmonary angiography. Radiol Case Rep 2022;17(11):4183–7. Published 2022 Sep 7.
28. Maruyama T, Kariya S, Nakatani M, et al. Congenital pulmonary varix: Two case reports. Medicine (Baltimore) 2021;100(51):e28340.

Neonatal and Pediatric Pulmonary Vascular Disease

Aki Tanimoto, MD*, R. Paul Guillerman, MD, Eric Crotty, MD, Andrew Schapiro, MD

KEYWORDS

- Pediatric imaging
- Pulmonary vascular disease
- Computed tomography
- MR imaging

KEY POINTS

- Children can be affected by a wide range of pulmonary vascular diseases, some of which present in infancy and others of which present later in childhood or adolescence.
- Some diseases present differently in children than adults due to disease heterogeneity, while others may present similarly in children and adults.
- Contrast enhanced computed tomography and magnetic resonance angiography provide detailed depiction of pediatric pulmonary vascular diseases.

INTRODUCTION

A wide spectrum of pulmonary vascular disorders causes considerable morbidity and mortality in the pediatric population. These disorders may present soon after birth or later in childhood or adolescence. Some of these disorders manifest similarly as in adults, while others are unique to neonates or children or have a much stronger association with genetic variants compared to adults. Anatomically, these disorders may primarily affect either the large pulmonary arteries or veins and be amenable to confident diagnosis by chest computed tomography (CT) or MR imaging angiography or involve the microvasculature at the level of the arterioles, venules, or capillaries with the imaging findings dependent on the secondary effects such as pulmonary hypertension, edema, or hemorrhage. Manifestations of these disorders can be restricted to the cardiopulmonary structures or associated with systemic diseases, syndromes, or anomalies in other body regions that serve as diagnostic clues. Although definitive diagnosis of some of these disorders depends on genetic testing or lung biopsy, appropriate imaging technique and knowledge of the characteristic imaging features of these disorders are essential to facilitate prompt diagnosis and guide clinical management.

LARGE PULMONARY VESSEL DEVELOPMENTAL ANOMALIES

Total Anomalous Pulmonary Venous Return/Partial Anomalous Pulmonary Venous Return and Scimitar Syndrome

Anomalous pulmonary venous return encompasses a spectrum of abnormal pulmonary venous connections in which at least 1 pulmonary vein drains outside of the left atrium. This results in an extracardiac left-to-right shunt. Total anomalous pulmonary venous return (TAPVR) requires a right-to-left shunt for survival via an atrial or ventricular septal defect, or patent ductus arteriosus. The 4 types of TAPVR classified based on the level of drainage include supracardiac, cardiac, infracardiac, and mixed types.[1] Anomalous drainage via a vertical vein into the left brachiocephalic vein is most commonly

Department of Radiology, Cincinnati Children's Hospital Medical Center, 3333 Burnet Avenue, Cincinnati, OH 45229, USA
* Corresponding author.
E-mail address: aki.tanimoto@cchmc.org

encountered.[2,3] Poorer prognosis after TAPVR repair is highest in neonatal patients, patients with preoperative pulmonary venous obstruction, and in infracardiac and mixed types.[1,4] Computed tomography angiography (CTA) plays an important role in the preoperative morphologic evaluation of TAPVR (Fig. 1A, B).

Patients with partial anomalous pulmonary venous return (PAPVR) do not typically exhibit symptoms in infancy and childhood,[5,6] and PAPVR is further discussed in Phan and colleagues' article, "Congenital Pulmonary Vascular Anomalies and Disease," in this issue. Scimitar syndrome is a rare congenital anomaly with a constellation of abnormalities including PAPVR and varying degrees of hypoplasia of the right lung and right pulmonary artery. Infantile presentation is most severe, with patients more likely to have aortopulmonary collaterals, congenital heart defects, pulmonary hypertension, non-cardiac anomalies, and higher rates of mortality than those presenting in childhood.[7–9] Childhood presentation typically manifests with recurrent pneumonia, murmur, and less significant associated defects.[8] Typical radiographic findings include hypoplastic right lung and dextroposition of the heart. The anomalous vein may be visible on chest radiography but is better delineated on CTA (Fig. 2A, B).

Pulmonary Sling

Pulmonary sling is a congenital vascular anomaly with an aberrant left pulmonary artery arising from the right pulmonary artery that courses between the trachea and esophagus to the left lung. Type 1 pulmonary slings are less common and usually associated with tracheobronchomalacia, but normal bronchial branching.[10,11] Type 2 slings are more common and associated with malformations of the tracheobronchial tree, particularly tracheal stenosis due to complete cartilaginous rings.[10,11] As a result of associated tracheobronchial abnormalities, most patients demonstrate signs and symptoms in the first year of life, including wheezing, dyspnea, and stridor.[12,13] While chest radiographs may give clues to tracheobronchial abnormalities, including a low T-shaped carina and asymmetric lung hyperinflation,[10,11,14] CTA is preferred for clear delineation of the pulmonary arteries and tracheobronchial anatomy (Fig. 3A, B).

Pulmonary Atresia

Pulmonary atresia is a congenital anomaly with lack of continuity between the right ventricle (RV) and pulmonary arteries with or without a ventricular septal defect. Pulmonary atresia with ventricular septal defect represents the most severe form of Tetralogy of Fallot. Pulmonary arterial supply is from systemic arterial circulation via a patent ductus arteriosus (PDA) and/or major aortopulmonary collateral arteries (MAPCAs), typically from the descending aorta.[15–17] While MAPCAs and a PDA can co-exist, they will not supply the same lung.[16] Those with ductal supply of the pulmonary arterial system typically present with normal distribution of the intrapulmonary arterial tree, whereas those with MAPCAs frequently demonstrate arborization abnormalities.[16] CTA accurately characterizes the branch pulmonary artery anatomy and pulmonary

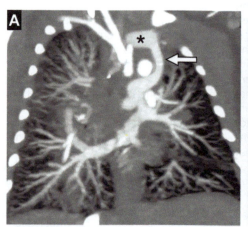
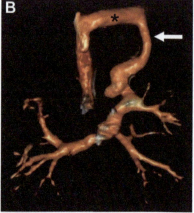

Fig. 1. A 0-day-old female with prenatally diagnosed supracardiac total anomalous pulmonary venous return (TAPVR). (*A*) Oblique coronal computed tomography (CT) with contrast shows connection of the 2 left pulmonary veins and the right lower pulmonary vein into a tortuous vertical vein (*white arrow*) that drains into the left brachiocephalic vein (*asterisk*). Right upper and middle pulmonary veins course medially toward the hilum without connection to the vertical draining vein, superior vena cava (SVC), or inferior vena cava (IVC). (*B*) Volume rendering of TAPVR.

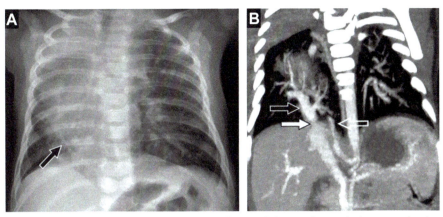

Fig. 2. An 11-week-old female with scimitar syndrome. (*A*) Frontal chest radiograph demonstrates dextroposition of the heart, scimitar vein (*black arrow*), hypoplastic right lung, and right upper lobe atelectasis. (*B*) Obliqued coronal CT image with contrast demonstrates anomalous right pulmonary venous drainage (*black arrow*) into the IVC with stenosis at the drainage site (*white arrow*). Anomalous systemic arterial supply to the right lower lobe from the abdominal aorta is also seen (*clear arrow*).

arterial blood supply necessary for surgical planning. Pulmonary atresia with intact interventricular septum presents with varying degrees of RV hypoplasia and hypertrophy, and frequent coronary anomalies.[18–20] Patients presenting with a thin and dilated RV and massively dilated right atrium demonstrate significant tricuspid regurgitation.[20,21] Those with significant hypertrophy and hypoplasia of the RV have hypoplastic tricuspid valves and egress of blood from the RV through ventriculo-coronary connections (sinusoids) thought to occur due to elevated RV pressure during development.[20–22] Notably, because blood flow to the pulmonary arteries is dependent on a PDA, MAPCAs are rarely present.[20] CTA can be used to delineate sinusoids, assess for coronary arterial stenosis or atresia, and define pulmonary arterial anatomy.[23]

Proximal Interruption of the Pulmonary Artery

Proximal interruption of the pulmonary artery (PIPA) is a rare congenital anomaly with an absent or blind-ending mediastinal portion of the pulmonary artery and normally developed intrapulmonary pulmonary arteries. Pulmonary arterial supply is through collaterals from bronchial arteries and transpleural branches of the intercostal, internal mammary, subclavian, or brachiocephalic arteries.[24] Most patients develop symptoms related to PIPA including recurrent pulmonary infections, hemoptysis, dyspnea, and pulmonary hypertension.[25–27] Early detection of PIPA is important as it may offer the opportunity for surgical repair. Radiographic findings include unilateral absence of normal hilar vascular density, decreased pulmonary

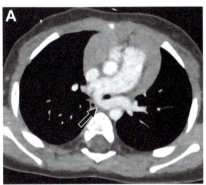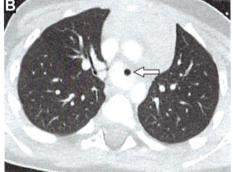

Fig. 3. A 10-month-old with murmur on examination diagnosed with pulmonary sling by CT. (*A*) Axial CT image with contrast demonstrates left pulmonary arterial sling (*black arrow*) with associated compression/narrowing of the distal thoracic trachea. (*B*) Axial CT image with contrast slightly superior to the main pulmonary artery demonstrates small caliber and round contour of the thoracic trachea (*white arrow*), consistent with complete tracheal rings.

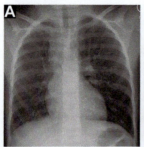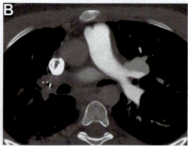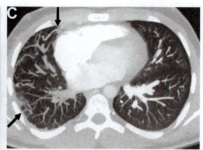

Fig. 4. Right-sided proximal interruption of the pulmonary artery (PIPA). (A) Frontal chest radiograph taken when patient was 9 year old demonstrates asymmetrically smaller right hemithorax with absence of the normal right hilar vascularity and peripheral reticulation predominantly at the right lung base. (B, C) CT obtained at 15 years of age demonstrates absent right pulmonary artery and numerous transpleural vessels supplying the right lung (black arrows).

vascular markings, and mild hypoplasia of the affected lung with mediastinal shift to the affected side.[24,28] On CT, the abnormal pulmonary artery terminates within 1 cm of its origin from the main pulmonary artery (Fig. 4A–C).

PULMONARY HYPERTENSION

Pulmonary arterial pressure equals systemic arterial pressure in utero, but falls rapidly after birth, reaching adult values by 3 months.[29] After 3 months of age, pulmonary hypertension (PH) is defined as a mean pulmonary arterial pressure of greater than 20 mm Hg, a definition established at the 6th World Symposium on Pulmonary Hypertension (WSPH) and adopted by the Pediatric Task Force of the 6th WSPH[30–33]

PH in children can begin at any age and as in adults can be due to many different etiologies. However, the distribution of PH etiologies in children is substantially different than in adults, with a greater predominance of idiopathic pulmonary arterial hypertension (PAH) as well as PH due to congenital heart disease (CHD) and developmental lung disease, and individual cases of PH in children are often associated with multiple etiologies.[31,34] In children, PH is currently classified according to the classification system established at the 6th WSPH.[30] Children with PH have a high prevalence of genetic disorders. For example, variants in the TBX4 gene are associated with neonatal diffuse developmental lung disorders, familial or sporadic childhood PAH, and small patella syndrome[35] (Fig. 5). Additional genetic disorders resulting in PAH are described in the following sections.

CT and cardiac MR imaging are important in the initial work-up of children with suspected PH.[36,37] CT is useful to assess for causes of secondary PH including vascular abnormalities, chronic thromboembolic disease, and parenchymal lung disease such as bronchopulmonary dysplasia (the most common lung disease associated with PH in children) (Fig. 6A, B).[33,36,38,39] Cardiac MR imaging is useful to assess cardiac morphology and function. Nuclear medicine ventilation-perfusion imaging is also sometimes used to evaluate for evidence of chronic thromboembolic pulmonary hypertension.[36,40]

PULMONARY VASCULAR DISEASE ASSOCIATED WITH GENETIC CONDITIONS
Williams Syndrome

Williams syndrome is an autosomal dominant syndrome typically associated with a de novo chromosome 7q11.23 deletion encompassing the ELN gene that encodes the protein elastin. In addition to cognitive impairment, distinctive "elfin"

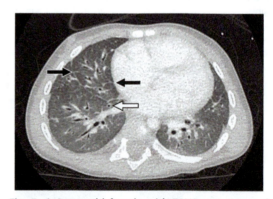

Fig. 5. A 1-year-old female with TBX4 mutation and pulmonary hypertension. Axial chest CT image with contrast shows diffuse ground-glass opacity, scattered interlobular septal thickening (black arrows), and bronchial wall thickening (white arrow) suggesting diffuse lung disease. Lung biopsy performed 2 years later demonstrated diffuse and marked interstitial chronic inflammation and fibrosis with lobular remodeling.

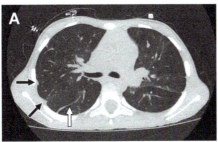 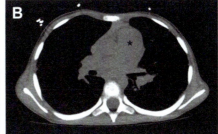

Fig. 6. An 11-year-old male with history of bronchopulmonary dysplasia (BPD) and pulmonary hypertension. (*A*) Axial chest CT image without contrast shows mosaic attenuation, pleural irregularity (*black arrows*), and a band-like opacity (*white arrow*) typical of patients with history of BPD. (*B*) Axial chest CT image without contrast shows an enlarged main pulmonary artery (*asterisk*).

facial features, and hypercalcemia in infancy, the syndrome is associated with cardiovascular abnormalities including supravalvular aortic stenosis and peripheral or branch pulmonary artery stenosis related to deficient circumferential arterial growth. Pulmonary artery stenosis occurs in approximately 60% of patients presenting in the first year of life and may be amenable to surgical pulmonary artery reconstruction but tends to progressively improve with age (**Fig. 7**A–D).[32] Pulmonary arterial diverticula at the bifurcation of the main pulmonary artery may also be observed.[33]

Alagille Syndrome

Alagille syndrome is an autosomal dominant syndrome caused by mutations in the *JAG1* gene encoding the Jagged 1 ligand in the Notch

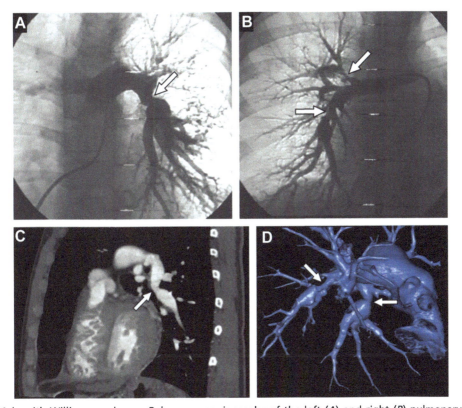

Fig. 7. Male with Williams syndrome. Pulmonary angiography of the left (*A*) and right (*B*) pulmonary arteries from when the patient was 13 year old as well as sagittal chest computed tomography angiography (CTA) image with contrast of the left pulmonary arteries (*C*) and 3-dimensional (3D) volume rendering of the pulmonary arterial system (*D*) from when the patient was 34 year old showing pulmonary artery stenosis (*white arrows*).

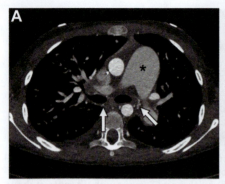
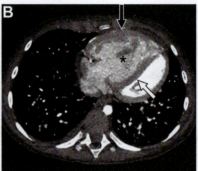
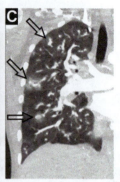

Fig. 8. An 11-year-old male with SOX17 mutation and severe pulmonary hypertension. (A) Axial CT image with contrast showing dilation of the main pulmonary artery (*asterisk*) and dilated bronchial arteries (*white arrows*). (B) Axial CT image with contrast showing right ventricular enlargement (*asterisk*) and myocardial thickening (*black arrow*) as well as leftward bowing of the interventricular septum (*white arrow*). (C) Coronal CT image with contrast showing ground-glass halos around pulmonary arteries (clear *arrows*).

signaling pathway, resulting in bile duct paucity, butterfly vertebrae, ocular and cardiovascular abnormalities, most commonly pulmonary artery stenosis. On CTA, the stenoses most often involve the proximal left pulmonary artery and lobar and segmental pulmonary artery branch points.[41] Associated congenital heart disease, most commonly tetralogy of Fallot, is associated with increased morbidity and mortality.[42]

BMPR2-Associated Familial Pulmonary Arterial Hypertension

Germline mutations of the *BMPR2* gene encoding the bone morphogenetic protein receptor type 2 transforming growth factor beta receptor are the predominant cause of familial PAH. Altered receptor signaling induces proliferation of smooth muscle cells and apoptosis-resistant endothelial cell clones in small pulmonary arteries, resulting in plexiform lesions at pulmonary arterial branchpoints and the origin of supernumerary vessels, appearing as ground-glass nodules with a central vessel on CT.[43] These plexiform lesions are not pathognomonic of *BMPR2*-associated familial PAH, and can also be observed in idiopathic PAH and in PAH in the setting of interstitial lung disease or congenital heart disease associated with low levels of *BMPR2* expression or signaling.[44]

SOX17-Associated Pulmonary Arterial Hypertension

Autosomal dominant mutations in the *SOX17* gene that encode SRY-box 17 involved in pulmonary vasculature formation and homeostasis are associated with severe sporadic or familial PAH. The PAH can be associated with life-threatening hemoptysis and cardiac septal defects, especially in young children. CT findings include dilated and tortuous pulmonary arteries, ground-glass halos around pulmonary arteries, and dilated bronchial arteries and subpleural vessels (**Fig. 8**A–C).[45]

Hereditary Hemorrhagic Telangiectasia

Hereditary hemorrhagic telangiectasia (HHT) is associated with pulmonary, hepatic, gastrointestinal, cerebrospinal, and mucocutaneous arteriovenous malformations (AVMs). Several genes have been implicated in the pathogenesis of HHT, including *ENG, ACVRL1 (ALK1), SMAD4, HHT3* and *HHT4*. On CT, pulmonary AVMs classically appear as an enhancing vascular tangle with feeding and draining vessels that may be amenable to endovascular therapy, although tiny

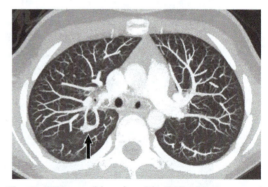

Fig. 9. A 9-year-old male with *ENG*-mutation-associated hereditary hemorrhagic telangiectasia, dyspnea with exertion, and positive bubble echocardiography. Axial maximum intensity projection chest CT image with contrast shows a right pulmonary arteriovenous malformation (*black arrow*).

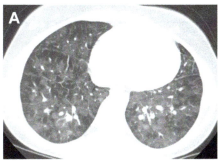 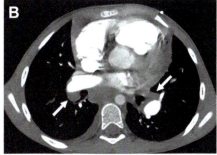

Fig. 10. An 18-year-old female with pulmonary hypertension from pulmonary veno-occlusive disease. (A) Axial chest CT image with contrast shows interlobular septal thickening and ground-glass opacities. (B) Axial chest CT image with contrast reveals hilar lymph node enlargement.

AVMs may appear as solid or ground-glass nodules (Fig. 9).[46] In the setting of *ACVRL1* mutations, PAH often precedes the manifestations of HHT.[47]

Pulmonary Veno-Occlusive Disease

Pulmonary veno-occlusive disease (PVOD) is a disorder associated with severe progressive PH due to increased pulmonary vascular resistance from pulmonary venule wall thickening, occlusion, and capillary proliferation. Cases may be sporadic, related to toxic exposure, or familial with mutations in the eukaryotic translation initiation factor 2 alpha kinase 4 (*EIF2AK4*) gene. Distinction of PVOD from PAH is critical for guiding appropriate management as pulmonary arterial vasodilators can induce life-threatening pulmonary edema in PVOD patients. PVOD has a more rapid deleterious course than PAH, and lung transplantation is the only treatment offering long-term survival.[36] Characteristic findings of childhood PVOD include interlobular septal thickening, poorly defined centrilobular ground-glass opacities, and lymphadenopathy[37,40] (Fig. 10A, B).

PULMONARY THROMBOEMBOLIC DISEASE

Pulmonary thromboembolism (PE) has historically been rarely diagnosed in children compared to adults. Unlike in adults, venous thromboembolic disease is rarely idiopathic in pediatric patients, with most patients having other serious associated conditions including cancer, congenital heart disease, and nephrotic syndrome.[38,39] Prior studies have demonstrated that the presence of a central venous catheter (CVC) is the single most important predisposing cause of deep venous thrombosis (DVT) in children.[38,39,48] One study found that nearly two-thirds of DVTs were detected in the upper extremities in the setting of a CVC.[39] The same study demonstrated that 56% of PE was CVC-related, with concurrent DVTs also found outside of the pulmonary arterial tree.[39] The ages of greatest risk for venous thromboembolism are infants less than 1 year of age and teenagers.[39,49] Given the potential morbidity and mortality associated with PE and non-specific clinical signs and symptoms, imaging studies play a critical role in the diagnosis of PE.[50,51]

Evaluation for PE may be performed with nuclear medicine lung ventilation-perfusion scintigraphy (V/Q scan), which offers low radiation exposure. However, it is notable that a "low probability" V/Q scan still carries a 20% chance of PE.[50] The current imaging modality of choice for pediatric PE evaluation is pulmonary CTA due its high spatial and contrast resolution, rapid imaging time, high sensitivity and specificity, and wide availability.

Table 1		
Vasculitides involving the pulmonary vasculature		
Predominantly Large Vessel Vasculitis	Predominantly Small Vessel Vasculitis	Other Vasculitides
Takayasu arteritis	Granulomatosis with polyangiitis Eosinophilic granulomatosis with polyangiitis Microscopic polyangiitis COPA syndrome Henoch-Schönlein purpura	Behçet disease Vasculitis associated with connective tissue diseases

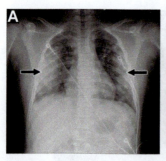 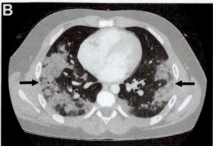 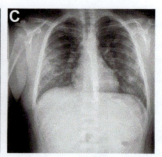

Fig. 11. A 12-year-old male with recently diagnosed Henoch-Schönlein purpura in the setting of lower extremity purpura, now presenting with hemoptysis. (*A*) Anteroposterior chest radiograph shows bilateral peripheral opacities (*black arrows*). (*B*) Axial chest CT image with contrast shows bilateral peripheral ground-glass opacity and consolidation (*black arrows*) compatible with hemorrhage. (*C*) Posteroanterior chest radiograph obtained 3 days later shows substantial decrease in bilateral lung opacities compatible with resolving hemorrhage.

PULMONARY VASCULAR DISEASE ASSOCIATED WITH SYSTEMIC AUTOIMMUNE CONDITIONS
Vasculitis

Pediatric vasculitides were classified by the European League Against Rheumatism and Pediatric Rheumatology European Society in 2005 according to the size of the predominantly involved vessels.[52] Some of these vasculitides can involve the pulmonary vasculature (**Table 1**). The larger pulmonary arteries can be involved in Takayasu arteritis and Behçet disease, with stenoses and occlusions typically seen with the former and aneurysms, occlusions, and thromboses potentially seen with the latter.[53,54] Imaging findings of small vessel vasculitides include nodules and masses, sometimes with cavitation, and areas of ground-glass opacity and consolidation, often reflecting pulmonary hemorrhage (**Fig. 11**A–C).[54–59] Although these findings alone are nonspecific, additional imaging findings and clinical history may help with the diagnosis. For instance, associated tracheobronchial stenosis suggests granulomatosis with polyangiitis; asthma and/or peripheral eosinophilia raises concern for eosinophilic granulomatosis with polyangiitis, lower extremity predominant purpura raises concern for Henoch-Schönlein purpura, and oral and genital ulcers raises concern for Behçet disease.[60–62] Early childhood diffuse alveolar hemorrhage, arthritis in adolescence, or a family history of these conditions raises concern for COPA syndrome (**Fig. 12**).[63]

Connective Tissue Disease-Associated Vasculopathy

Connective tissue disease-associated pulmonary vascular disease can occur in children with juvenile systemic sclerosis (SSc), mixed connective tissue disease (MCTD), systemic lupus erythematosus (SLE), and systemic juvenile idiopathic arthritis (sJIA). Although less common in children than in adults, pulmonary arterial hypertension can occur in children with SSc and MCTD and is associated with a poor prognosis.[64–67] In SLE, PAH, PE, and diffuse alveolar hemorrhage can all rarely occur. In patients with sJIA-associated lung disease, arterial wall thickening is often seen at histopathology and can be associated with PAH.[68–70]

MISCELLANEOUS ACQUIRED PULMONARY VASCULAR DISEASES
Pulmonary Vein Stenosis

Pulmonary vein stenosis (PVS) is an under recognized condition associated with PH and high mortality that most often occurs in newborns and infants with prematurity, bronchopulmonary dysplasia (BPD), and CHD. PVS may be primary or secondary. Primary PVS usually presents in mid-late infancy with age at presentation and severity of symptoms related to the number of veins involved and the degree of narrowing.

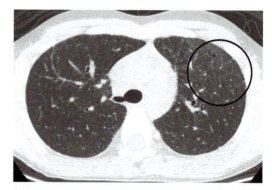

Fig. 12. A 7-year-old female with COPA syndrome. Axial chest CT image without contrast demonstrates left upper lobe ground-glass opacities, interlobular septal thickening, and tiny cysts (*circle*) related to recurrent pulmonary hemorrhage and fibrosis.

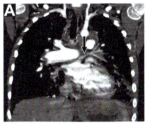 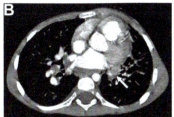 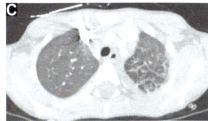

Fig. 13. A 4-year-old male with pulmonary vein stenosis (PVS). (*A*) Coronal chest computed tomography angiography (CTA) image with contrast shows a small caliber left upper pulmonary vein (*black arrow*). (*B*) Axial chest CTA image with contrast demonstrates left hilar soft tissue (*white arrow*). (*C*) Axial chest CT image with contrast shows left upper lobe interlobular septal thickening representing interstitial pulmonary edema from PVS.

Primary PVS has a poor prognosis, typically presenting with progressive stenosis and with restenosis following therapy. The involved segment is usually focally narrowed, but may involve a longer segment, or the veins may be diffusely small.[71] Secondary PVS occurs in children with prior surgical intervention, especially following repair of TAPVR/PAPVR. Primary and secondary PVS most commonly occurs at the atrial insertion site.

Echocardiography is most commonly used for diagnosis and follow-up of PVS, but can be falsely negative in approximately 25% of cases.[72] Increasingly, CTA is used as the modality of choice for confirmation. CTA has high specificity but limited sensitivity for PVS, so conventional angiography should be considered if there is high clinical suspicion in the setting of a negative CTA.[73] Focal ground-glass opacity, interlobular septal thickening, and hilar soft tissue are ancillary CT findings strongly associated with ipsilateral PVS that assist in distinction from chronic lung disease of prematurity[74] (**Fig. 13**A–C). MR imaging may also be used to evaluate the extent of a stenotic vein and can quantify differential blood flow,[75] but is limited by spatial resolution and more often requires sedation. Nuclear medicine lung perfusion imaging is an excellent method for evaluating regional perfusion abnormalities including evaluating the response to therapy.[76]

Hepatopulmonary Syndrome

Hepatopulmonary syndrome occurs when patients with advanced hepatic dysfunction develop dilation of precapillary and capillary vessels, and the resultant increased alveolar-arterial oxygen gradient leads to hypoxemia.[77] The same physiology is also seen in patients with deficient flow of hepatic venous blood to the lungs as occurs in patients with extrahepatic portosystemic shunts (Abernethy syndrome) and certain cavopulmonary shunts.[78] By a yet unknown mechanism, this results in dilation of peripheral pulmonary arterial branches and rapid intrapulmonary transit of pulmonary arterial blood to the pulmonary veins. Diffuse microscopic pulmonary arteriovenous malformations (pAVMs) can also develop.[79]

Imaging usually commences with microbubble/contrast-enhanced echocardiography, where the rapid transit time manifests as quicker than expected return of the microbubbles to the left atrium.[80] CT shows dilation of the pulmonary arterial branches, which can be seen extending to the pleural surface, especially in the lower lobes[81] (**Fig. 14**). Less commonly seen is nodular dilation

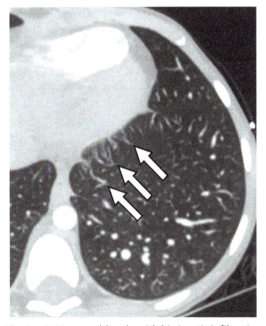

Fig. 14. A 10-year-old male with histiocytic infiltration of the liver and resultant liver impairment, presenting with dyspnea and hypoxia. Bubble echocardiography was positive for intrapulmonary shunting. Axial CT image with contrast demonstrates dilated peripheral pulmonary vessels extending to the pleura (*white arrows*).

of the subpleural pulmonary vessels, representing the microscopic pAVMs.[82] These findings have been seen to resolve or regress substantially after liver transplantation, conversion to a total cavopulmonary anastomosis in children with superior cavopulmonary/Glenn anastomosis, and after redirection of hepatic venous blood to the pulmonary arterial tree in patients with a prior Kawashima procedure[77,78]

SUMMARY

Children can be affected by a broad range of pulmonary vascular diseases. While disorders such as pulmonary thromboembolism and pulmonary hypertension appear similar on imaging in children and adults, the underlying predisposing conditions vary across age groups, and some diseases manifest predominantly in infancy, in particular certain congenital anomalies and genetic disorders. Recognition of extrapulmonary findings assists the diagnosis of syndromic and systemic disorders, such as butterfly vertebrae in Alagille syndrome, small patellae in *TBX4*-associated PAH, and arthritis in COPA syndrome. Chest CT and MR imaging angiography techniques can directly depict diseases involving the large and medium-sized pulmonary vessels, while the imaging findings of small vessel vasculitis, PVOD, and other diseases involving the microvasculature are dependent on secondary effects such as pulmonary hypertension, edema, or hemorrhage. Knowledge of the characteristic imaging features of these diseases is essential to facilitate prompt diagnosis and guide clinical management.

CLINICS CARE POINTS

- Developmental anomalies of the pulmonary vasculature can be clearly delineated with CT and magnetic resonance to aid in surgical planning.
- Pediatric PH presents similarly to adults, but the distribution of etiologies is substantially different in children, with a greater proportion of cases due to CHD, developmental lung disease, and certain genetic conditions
- Numerous genetic conditions result in pulmonary vascular disease, and are often associated with additional findings that can help suggest diagnosis
- Pulmonary embolism is less common in pediatric patients than in adults, and the distribution of associated DVT tends to be in the upper extremities.
- Autoimmune diseases, including vasculitides and connective tissue disorders, affect the pulmonary vasculature of pediatric patients, similar to adults.

DISCLOSURE

The authors do not have any relevant disclosures.

FUNDING

A. Tanimoto received supporting funding from the Society for Pediatric Radiology Research and Education Foundation William H. and Victoria McAlister Young Investigator Award. There are no external funding sources to report for the other authors.

REFERENCES

1. Karamlou T, Gurofsky R, Al Sukhni E, et al. Factors associated with mortality and reoperation in 377 children with total anomalous pulmonary venous connection. Circulation 2007;115(12):1591–8.
2. Burroughs JT, Edwards JE. Total anomalous pulmonary venous connection. Am Heart J 1960;59(6):913–31.
3. Gathman GE, Nadas AS. Total anomalous pulmonary venous connection. Circulation 1970;42(1):143–54.
4. Shi G, Zhu Z, Chen J, et al. Total anomalous pulmonary venous connection: the current management strategies in a pediatric cohort of 768 patients. Circulation 2017;135(1):48–58.
5. Senocak F, Ozme S, Bilgiç A, et al. Partial anomalous pulmonary venous return. Evaluation of 51 cases. Jpn Heart J 1994;35(1):43–50.
6. Hijii T, Fukushige J, Hara T. Diagnosis and management of partial anomalous pulmonary venous connection. A review of 28 pediatric cases. Cardiology 1998;89(2):148–51.
7. Seymour E, Mallory G, Morales-Demori R. Surgical and cardiac catheterization outcomes of scimitar syndrome patients: a three decade single-center experience. Pediatr Cardiol 2023;44(3):579–86.
8. Canter CE, Martin TC, Spray TL, et al. Scimitar syndrome in childhood. Am J Cardiol 1986;58(7):652–4.
9. Huddleston CB, Exil V, Canter CE, et al. Scimitar syndrome presenting in infancy. Ann Thorac Surg 1999;67(1):154–9.
10. Newman B, Cho Y ah. Left pulmonary artery sling-anatomy and imaging. Semin Ultrasound CT MRI 2010;31(2):158–70.
11. Wells TR, Gwinn JL, Landing BH, et al. Reconsideration of the anatomy of sling left pulmonary artery: the association of one form with bridging bronchus

and imperforate anus. Anatomic and diagnostic aspects. J Pediatr Surg 1988;23(10):892–8.
12. Lee KH, Yoon CS, Choe KO, et al. Use of imaging for assessing anatomical relationships of tracheobronchial anomalies associated with left pulmonary artery sling. Pediatr Radiol 2001;31(4):269–78.
13. Gikonyo BM, Jue KL, Edwards JE. Pulmonary vascular sling: report of seven cases and review of the literature. Pediatr Cardiol 1989;10(2):81–9.
14. Berdon WE. Rings, slings, and other things: vascular compression of the infant trachea updated from the midcentury to the millennium—the legacy of Robert E. Gross, MD, and Edward B. D. Neuhauser, MD. Radiology 2000;216(3):624–32.
15. Alex A, Ayyappan A, Valakkada J, et al. Major aortopulmonary collateral arteries. Radiol Cardiothorac Imaging. 2022;4(1):e210157.
16. Liao PK, Edwards WD, Julsrud PR, et al. Pulmonary blood supply in patients with pulmonary atresia and ventricular septal defect. J Am Coll Cardiol 1985; 6(6):1343–50.
17. Murthy K, Reddy KP, Nagarajan R, et al. Management of ventricular septal defect with pulmonary atresia and major aorto pulmonary collateral arteries: challenges and controversies. Ann Pediatr Cardiol 2010;3(2):127–35.
18. Bull C, de Leval MR, Mercanti C, et al. Pulmonary atresia and intact ventricular septum: a revised classification. Circulation 1982;66(2):266–72.
19. Alwi M. Management algorithm in pulmonary atresia with intact ventricular septum. Catheter Cardiovasc Interv 2006;67(5):679–86.
20. Daubeney PEF, Delany DJ, Anderson RH, et al. Pulmonary atresia with intact ventricular septum. J Am Coll Cardiol 2002;39(10):1670–9.
21. Chikkabyrappa SM, Loomba RS, Tretter JT. Pulmonary atresia with an intact ventricular septum: preoperative physiology, imaging, and management. Semin Cardiothorac Vasc Anesth 2018;22(3):245–55.
22. Freedom RM, Anderson RH, Perrin D. The significance of ventriculo-coronary arterial connections in the setting of pulmonary atresia with an intact ventricular septum. Cardiol Young 2005;15(5):447–68.
23. Escalon JG, Browne LP, Bang TJ, et al. Congenital anomalies of the pulmonary arteries: an imaging overview. Br J Radiol 2019;92(1093):20180185.
24. Kieffer SA, Amplatz K, Anderson RC, et al. Proximal interruption of a pulmonary artery: roentgen features and surgical correction. Am J Roentgenol 1965; 95(3):592–7.
25. Bouros D, Pare P, Panagou P, et al. The varied manifestation of pulmonary artery agenesis in adulthood. Chest 1995;108(3):670–6.
26. Ryu DS, Spirn PW, Trotman-Dickenson B, et al. HRCT findings of proximal interruption of the right pulmonary artery. J Thorac Imaging 2004;19(3):171–5.
27. Jan Ten Harkel AD, Blom NA, Ottenkamp J. Isolated unilateral absence of a pulmonary artery: a case report and review of the literature. Chest 2002; 122(4):1471–7.
28. Apostolopoulou SC, Kelekis NL, Brountzos EN, et al. "Absent" pulmonary artery in one adult and five pediatric patients: imaging, embryology, and therapeutic implications. Am J Roentgenol 2002;179(5): 1253–60.
29. Goss KN, Everett AD, Mourani PM, et al. Addressing the challenges of phenotyping pediatric pulmonary vascular disease. Pulm Circ 2017;7(1):7–19.
30. Simonneau G, Montani D, Celermajer DS, et al. Haemodynamic definitions and updated clinical classification of pulmonary hypertension. Eur Respir J 2019;53(1). https://doi.org/10.1183/13993003.01913-2018.
31. Rosenzweig EB, Abman SH, Adatia I, et al. Paediatric pulmonary arterial hypertension: updates on definition, classification, diagnostics and management. Eur Respir J 2019;53(1). https://doi.org/10.1183/13993003.01916-2018.
32. Collins RTI. Cardiovascular disease in Williams syndrome. Curr Opin Pediatr 2018;30(5):609.
33. Ahmad Z, Vettukattil J. Pulmonary artery diverticulum: an angiographic marker for Williams syndrome. Pediatr Cardiol 2010;31(5):611–4.
34. del Cerro Marín MJ, Rotés AS, Ogando AR, et al. Assessing pulmonary hypertensive vascular disease in childhood. Data from the Spanish registry. Am J Respir Crit Care Med 2014;190(12):1421–9.
35. Neves da Silva HV, Weinman JP, Englund EK, et al. Computed tomographic findings in TBX4 mutation: a common cause of severe pulmonary artery hypertension in children. Pediatr Radiol 2024;54(2):199–207.
36. Solinas S, Boucly A, Beurnier A, et al. Diagnosis and management of pulmonary veno-occlusive disease. Expert Rev Respir Med 2023;17(8):635–49.
37. Berteloot L, Proisy M, Jais JP, et al. Idiopathic, heritable and veno-occlusive pulmonary arterial hypertension in childhood: computed tomography angiography features in the initial assessment of the disease. Pediatr Radiol 2019;49(5):575–85.
38. Andrew M, David M, Adams M, et al. Venous thromboembolic complications (VTE) in children: first analyses of the Canadian Registry of VTE. Blood 1994; 83(5):1251–7.
39. Monagle P, Adams M, Mahoney M, et al. Outcome of pediatric thromboembolic disease: a report from the Canadian childhood thrombophilia registry. Pediatr Res 2000;47(6):763–6.
40. Woerner C, Cutz E, Yoo SJ, et al. Pulmonary venoocclusive disease in childhood. Chest 2014;146(1): 167–74.
41. Rodriguez RM, Feinstein JA, Chan FP. CT-defined phenotype of pulmonary artery stenoses in Alagille syndrome. Pediatr Radiol 2016;46(8):1120–7.

42. Luong R, Feinstein JA, Ma M, et al. Outcomes in patients with Alagille syndrome and complex pulmonary artery disease. J Pediatr 2021;229:86–94.e4.
43. Weinman JP, Mong DA, Malone LJ, et al. Chest computed tomography findings of ground-glass nodules with enhancing central vessel/nodule in pediatric patients with BMPR2 mutations and plexogenic arteriopathy. Pediatr Radiol 2022;52(13):2549–56.
44. St. Croix CM, Steinhorn RH. New thoughts about the origin of plexiform lesions. Am J Respir Crit Care Med 2016;193(5):484–5.
45. Montani D, Lechartier B, Girerd B, et al. An emerging phenotype of pulmonary arterial hypertension patients carrying SOX17 variants. Eur Respir J 2022;60(6):2200656.
46. Kolarich AR, Solomon AJ, Bailey C, et al. Imaging manifestations and interventional treatments for hereditary hemorrhagic telangiectasia. Radiographics 2021;41(7):2157–75.
47. Girerd B, Montani D, Coulet F, et al. Clinical Outcomes of pulmonary arterial hypertension in patients carrying an ACVRL1 (ALK1) mutation. Am J Respir Crit Care Med 2010;181(8):851–61.
48. van Ommen CH, Heijboer H, Büller HR, et al. Venous thromboembolism in childhood: a prospective two-year registry in The Netherlands. J Pediatr 2001;139(5):676–81.
49. Chan AK, Deveber G, Monagle P, et al. Venous thrombosis in children. J Thromb Haemost 2003;1(7):1443–55.
50. Victoria T, Mong A, Altes T, et al. Evaluation of pulmonary embolism in a pediatric population with high clinical suspicion. Pediatr Radiol 2009;39(1):35–41.
51. Thacker PG, Lee EY. Pulmonary embolism in children. Am J Roentgenol 2015;204(6):1278–88.
52. Ozen S, Ruperto N, Dillon MJ, et al. EULAR/PReS endorsed consensus criteria* for the classification of childhood vasculitides. Ann Rheum Dis 2006;65(7):936–41.
53. Sharma S, Kamalakar T, Rajani M, et al. The incidence and patterns of pulmonary artery involvement in takayasu's arteritis. Clin Radiol 1990;42(3):177–81.
54. Ceylan N, Bayraktaroglu S, Erturk SM, et al. Pulmonary and vascular manifestations of Behçet disease: imaging findings. Am J Roentgenol 2010;194(2):W158–64.
55. Khanna G, Sargar K, Baszis KW. Pediatric vasculitis: recognizing multisystemic manifestations at body imaging. Radiographics 2015;35(3):849–65.
56. Soliman M, Laxer R, Manson D, et al. Imaging of systemic vasculitis in childhood. Pediatr Radiol 2015;45(8):1110–25.
57. Worthy SA, Müller NL, Hansell DM, et al. Churg-Strauss syndrome: the spectrum of pulmonary CT findings in 17 patients. Am J Roentgenol 1998;170(2):297–300.
58. Connolly B, Manson D, Eberhard A, et al. CT appearance of pulmonary vasculitis in children. Am J Roentgenol 1996;167(4):901–4.
59. Di Pietro GM, Castellazzi ML, Mastrangelo A, et al. Henoch-Schönlein Purpura in children: not only kidney but also lung. Pediatr Rheumatol Online J 2019;17:75.
60. Ozen S, Pistorio A, Iusan SM, et al. EULAR/PRINTO/PRES criteria for Henoch–Schönlein purpura, childhood polyarteritis nodosa, childhood Wegener granulomatosis and childhood Takayasu arteritis: Ankara 2008. Part II: final classification criteria. Ann Rheum Dis 2010;69(5):798–806.
61. The American College of Rheumatology 1990 criteria for the classification of churg-strauss syndrome (allergic granulomatosis and angiitis) - Masi - 1990 - arthritis & Rheumatism - Wiley Online Library. Available at: https://onlinelibrary.wiley.com/doi/abs/10.1002/art.1780330806?sid=nlm%3Apubmed. Accessed August 8, 2024.
62. Koné-Paut I, Shahram F, Darce-Bello M, et al. Consensus classification criteria for paediatric Behçet's disease from a prospective observational cohort: PEDBD. Ann Rheum Dis 2016;75(6):958–64.
63. Nguyen HN, Salman R, Vogel TP, et al. Imaging findings of COPA syndrome. Pediatr Radiol 2023;53(5):844–53.
64. Rabinovich CE. Challenges in the diagnosis and treatment of juvenile systemic sclerosis. Nat Rev Rheumatol 2011;7(11):676–80.
65. Martini G, Foeldvari I, Russo R, et al. Systemic sclerosis in childhood: clinical and immunologic features of 153 patients in an international database. Arthritis Rheum 2006;54(12):3971–8.
66. Berard RA, Laxer RM. Pediatric mixed connective tissue disease. Curr Rheumatol Rep 2016;18(5):28.
67. Burdt MA, Hoffman RW, Deutscher SL, et al. Long-term outcome in mixed connective tissue disease: longitudinal clinical and serologic findings. Arthritis Rheum 1999;42(5):899–909.
68. Saper VE, Chen G, Deutsch GH, et al. Emergent high fatality lung disease in systemic juvenile arthritis. Ann Rheum Dis 2019;78(12):1722–31.
69. Schulert GS, Yasin S, Carey B, et al. Systemic juvenile idiopathic arthritis-lung disease: characterization and risk factors. Arthritis Rheumatol Hoboken NJ 2019;71(11):1943–54.
70. Palafox-Flores JG, Valencia-Ledezma OE, Vargas-López G, et al. Systemic lupus erythematosus in pediatric patients: pulmonary manifestations. Respir Med 2023;220:107456.
71. Romberg EK, Stanescu AL, Bhutta ST, et al. Computed tomography of pulmonary veins: review of congenital and acquired pathologies. Pediatr Radiol 2022;52(13):2510–28.

72. Seale AN, Webber SA, Uemura H, et al. Pulmonary vein stenosis: the UK, Ireland and Sweden collaborative study. Heart 2009;95(23):1944–9.
73. Barrera CA, Saul D, Rapp JB, et al. Diagnostic performance of CT angiography to detect pulmonary vein stenosis in children. Int J Cardiovasc Imaging 2020;36(1):141–7.
74. O'Callaghan B, Zablah JE, Weinman JP, et al. Computed tomographic parenchymal lung findings in premature infants with pulmonary vein stenosis. Pediatr Radiol 2023;53(9):1874–84.
75. Rito ML, Gazzaz T, Wilder TJ, et al. Pulmonary vein stenosis: severity and location predict survival after surgical repair. J Thorac Cardiovasc Surg 2016;151(3):657–66.e2.
76. Drubach LA, Jenkins KJ, Stamoulis C, et al. Evaluation of primary pulmonary vein stenosis in children: comparison of radionuclide perfusion lung scan and angiography. Am J Roentgenol 2015;205(4):873–7.
77. Krowka MJ, Fallon MB, Kawut SM, et al. International liver transplant Society Practice Guidelines: diagnosis and management of hepatopulmonary syndrome and portopulmonary hypertension. Transplantation 2016;100(7):1440.
78. Alibrahim IJ, Mohammed MHA, Kabbani MS, et al. Pulmonary arteriovenous malformations in children after the Kawashima procedure: risk factors and midterm outcome. Ann Pediatr Cardiol 2021;14(1):10.
79. McFaul RC, Tajik AJ, Mair DD, et al. Development of pulmonary arteriovenous shunt after superior vena cava-right pulmonary artery (Glenn) anastomosis. Report of four cases. Circulation 1977;55(1):212–6.
80. Gudavalli A, Kalaria VG, Chen X, et al. Intrapulmonary arteriovenous shunt: diagnosis by saline contrast bubbles in the pulmonary veins. J Am Soc Echocardiogr 2002;15(9):1012–4.
81. McAdams HP, Erasmus J, Crockett R, et al. The hepatopulmonary syndrome: radiologic findings in 10 patients. Am J Roentgenol 1996;166(6):1379–85.
82. Krowka MJ, Dickson ER, Cortese DA. Hepatopulmonary syndrome: clinical observations and lack of therapeutic response to somatostatin analogue. Chest 1993;104(2):515–21.

Role of Cardiovascular MR Imaging and MR Angiography in Patients with Pulmonary Vascular Disease

Tugce Agirlar Trabzonlu, MD, Bradley D. Allen, MD*

KEYWORDS

- MR pulmonary angiography • MR perfusion • MR imaging of pulmonary embolism
- Pulmonary hypertension

KEY POINTS

- Pulmonary MR angiography (MRA) is a feasible imaging alternative to computed tomography angiography (CTA) in pulmonary embolism detection.
- Perfusion MR imaging and cardiac MR imaging help diagnose and monitor the treatment response of chronic thromboembolic pulmonary hypertension.
- Cardiac MR imaging is pivotal in assessing the potential underlying etiology and impact of pulmonary hypertension on the heart by providing reference-standard noninvasive cardiac morphology and function assessment and tissue characterization.
- Multiphasic acquisitions and dynamic phase imaging are unique to pulmonary MRA, which aid in diagnosing many pulmonary vascular diseases, including shunts and masses.

 Video content accompanies this article at http://www.radiologic.theclinics.com.

INTRODUCTION

Pulmonary vascular diseases are an important cause of patient morbidity and mortality. Acute pulmonary embolism affects 1 in 1000 people annually and is the third most common cause of acute cardiovascular mortality.[1,2] Other pulmonary artery diseases include pulmonary hypertension, vasculitis, aneurysms, congenital diseases, arteriovenous malformations, shunts, and masses.[3] Computed tomographic (CT) pulmonary artery angiography is the reference standard for evaluating pulmonary vasculature with excellent resolution, wide availability, and fast acquisition.[2] Historically, MR pulmonary angiography had limited clinical use in evaluating pulmonary vascular disease. The limitations included low resolution and artifacts from slow flow, respiratory, and cardiac motion; resulting in low sensitivity and specificity.[1,4] However, MR pulmonary angiography has become a promising diagnostic tool with newly evolving techniques, wider availability, and faster acquisitions. In patients with moderate-to-severe iodinated contrast allergy and renal failure, MR angiography (MRA) may be a feasible diagnostic alternative in pulmonary embolism detection. In 2022, coronavirus disease 2019-related lockdowns resulted in a worldwide iodinated contrast media shortage where some centers used MR pulmonary angiography as a substitute for CTA to evaluate for pulmonary embolism.[5]

Radiology Department, Northwestern University Feinberg School of Medicine, Arkes Pavilion, 676 North St Clair Street, Suite 800, Chicago, IL 60611, USA
* Corresponding author.
E-mail addresses: tugce.agirlartrabzonlu@nm.org (T.A.T.); bdallen@northwestern.edu (B.D.A.)

Furthermore, lung perfusion MR imaging is a unique technique for perfusion assessment without the requirement for iodinated contrast or radiation exposure.[6] Cardiac MR imaging is the noninvasive reference standard imaging tool to assess cardiac morphology and function. It has a pivotal role in managing patients with pulmonary hypertension or other pulmonary vascular diseases.[7] Thus, when used alone or combined, MR pulmonary angiography, cardiac MR imaging, and perfusion MR imaging are essential in managing patients with pulmonary vascular disease.[2,4] This study reviews technique, limitations, and clinical applications of cardiovascular MR imaging and MRA in patients with pulmonary vascular disease.

IMAGING TECHNIQUE
Noncontrast MR Pulmonary Angiography

Balanced steady-state gradient echo sequence

The balanced steady-state free precession (bSSFP) sequences have been commercially available for over 20 years.[2] The steady-state free precession (SSFP) sequence provides high contrast of the blood pool with minimal flow dependency.[2] SSFP sequences obtained at axial, coronal, and sagittal planes may allow evaluation of central pulmonary embolism in fewer than 5 minutes of acquisition.[1] Heredia and colleagues demonstrated that SSFP imaging provides a good image quality in all central and lobar pulmonary artery branches and 90% of segmental pulmonary arteries.[8] Kaya and colleagues[9] demonstrated that the sensitivity of pulmonary embolism detection was 87.9% with SSFP sequences. Unlike spin echo sequences, SSFP is more susceptible to the B0 magnetic field inhomogeneities, resulting in off-resonance banding artifacts and low imaging quality of peripheral branches.[2] Thus, the SSFP sequences should be obtained when combined with subsequent contrast-enhanced sequences to confirm or increase the sensitivity and specificity of pulmonary embolism detection.

A navigator (NAV)-gated 3 dimensional (3D) SSFP imaging can provide rapid 3D imaging with free breathing and take approximately 3 minutes to obtain.[10] Hui and colleagues[10] showed that the NAV-gated SSFP images are comparable to the breath-hold SSFP sequences.

Three dimensional fresh blood imaging using 3 dimensional fast spin echo-based sequence

The 3D fast spin echo (FSE)-based sequence could provide 3D non-enhanced MRA or MR venography (MRV) imaging using electrocardiogram (ECG) gating. The sequence depends on differences in the blood flow during systole and diastole of the cardiac cycle. ECG-triggered imaging during diastole provides signals from arterial structures that have a relatively slow flow. MR imaging of the venous structures could be obtained similarly due to their constant slow flow. The images are moderate-to-heavily T2 weighted with this sequence.[2]

Contrast-enhanced MR Pulmonary Angiography

High-resolution 3 dimensional T1-weighted spoiled gradient echo

Contrast-enhanced MR angiography is the most accurate MRA technique in evaluating pulmonary arteries.[11] In this technique, the gadolinium-based contrast agent results in T1 shortening and high signal of the vasculature. The images are obtained with a very short relaxation time (TR) of less than 5 msec and an echo time (TE) of less than 2 msec; using a fast low-angle single shot (FLASH) technique.[12] A short TE prevents signal loss from inhomogeneous magnetic susceptibility from background lung parenchyma and reduces artifacts. A short TR enables imaging with shorter breath holds. The acquisition time can be further decreased by parallel imaging. The images are usually acquired in coronal plane to reduce the required number of slices for coverage. The arms-up position prevents wrap-around artifacts.[4,12]

The gadolinium-based contrast media is injected via a peripheral vein as a bolus with an automated power injector. A standard dose of gadolinium-based contrast (0.1 mmol/kg) is used with a flow rate of 2 to 5 mL/s to obtain an optimal bolus, which is followed by a 20 mL saline flush.[4] Acquisition at the optimal timing during the maximized pulmonary vascular signal intensity is critical. The contrast media concentration is adjusted to the central k-space acquisition timing. Nonoptimized imaging may preclude pulmonary arterial assessment due to suboptimal opacification of the pulmonary artery branches and opacification of the pulmonary veins.[4] The timing could be determined by care bolus/MR fluoroscopy technique or test bolus examination.[11] A series of delayed phase images can often be helpful in problem-solving, especially for bolus timing-related suboptimal opacification or artifacts.

Time-resolved MR Angiography

Time-resolved MRA (TR-MRA) provides rapid multiphasic imaging of the pulmonary vasculature, which benefits patients with severe dyspnea. With parallel imaging, the MRA images could be obtained in less than 10 seconds with a temporal resolution of 1 second.[2,11] Optimized bolus timing is not required as injection and image acquisition occur simultaneously.[4] Furthermore, pulmonary venous and aortic imaging could be obtained during the same session. TR-MRA is used to evaluate pulmonary venous anatomy for pre-procedural assessment of atrial fibrillation ablation, vascular shunts, arteriovenous malformation, and vascular anomalies.[12–14] During TR-MRA acquisition, there is relatively more frequent sampling of the center of the k-space than the periphery.[4,11] Thus, although the imaging has good contrast resolution, the evaluation of the peripheral branches may be degraded due to low spatial resolution.[13] A standard dose of gadolinium-based contrast (0.1 mL/kg) should be used with a high flow rate to obtain an optimal bolus.[2]

PITFALLS, LIMITATIONS, ARTIFACTS, AND HOW TO SOLVE THEM

Pulmonary MR imaging is difficult due to the heavily T2*-weighted signal of air (0.5 msec T2* at 1.5 T and 2 msec T2* at 3T).[1] Increased susceptibility limits the delineation of small peripheral vessels. These effects could be decreased by using a 1.5 T scanner, employing short TE GRE sequences, scanning during expiration, and parallel imaging.[1]

Maki artifact occurs due to inadequate timing of the contrast bolus relative to k-space sampling. If the contrast bolus arrives in the middle of the acquisition, the center of the k-space is obtained with minimal contrast in the pulmonary arteries, and the edges are obtained when contrast is present. This results in transient enhancement of the periphery of the vessel and signal drop of the center.[15] The artifact could be prevented by diluting the intravenous contrast and ensuring diluted contrast administration throughout the acquisition.[1] Obtaining a delayed phase in addition to the arterial phase can help distinguish artifact from a true embolism (**Fig. 1**A–C).[15]

Truncation artifact (Gibbs or ringing artifact) is seen near the abrupt transitions between regions of high and low signal intensity. The artifact results in central low signal intensity in pulmonary arteries 3 to 5 pixels in diameter, such as lobar or segmental pulmonary artery branches. Identification of this artifact is usually straightforward with experienced readers; however, it may be difficult for inexperienced radiologists. Bannas and colleagues[15] demonstrated that a signal drop with a cut-off value greater than 51% on the arterial phase and >47% on the delayed phase could distinguish artifact from pulmonary embolism with high sensitivity (100%) and specificity (>90%).

Additional MR imaging artifacts, such as motion and wrap around (aliasing), can occur. Careful selection of patients who can hold their breath is essential to avoid motion artifacts with pulmonary MRA. Having the patient raise their arms can avoid the wrap-around artifacts. The aliasing artifacts can be avoided by increasing the field of view, although this results in a longer breath-hold acquisition.

ADDITIONAL TECHNIQUES
Ferumoxytol as a Contrast Agent

Ferumoxytol (Feraheme, AMAG) is an ultrasmall superparamagnetic iron oxide particle approved by Food and Drug Administration for parenteral iron deficiency anemia treatment. It causes T1 shortening and can be an alternative MR contrast agent in patients with moderate-to-severe gadolinium contrast allergy. It has a relatively prolonged intravascular half-life of 15 hours, allowing repeat imaging in technically inadequate studies and same-session lower extremity MRV, as needed. The dose for MRA (3–4 mg/kg) is lower than for anemia treatment and requires a slow infusion rather than rapid bolus administration as it may cause side effects such as hypotension and death.[1,16] The acquisition time is short and requires a few breath holds.[16] The limitations of ferumoxytol are longer preparation time, requirement for slow infusion and monitoring after the infusion, transient signal alteration on subsequent MR imaging studies, and relatively high cost.[17] Starekova and colleagues.[16] showed that ferumoxytol-enhanced MRA provided a good or excellent image quality MR pulmonary angiography in pregnant patients in most cases.

MR Perfusion

Noncontrast MR pulmonary perfusion
Fourier decomposition techniques provide ventilation and perfusion images using differences in signal changes during inspiration and exhalation and cardiac systole and diastole. Arterial spin labeling provides perfusion maps by labeling the intrinsic contrast of magnetized inflowing flow. Currently, these methods do not have any clinical application due to artifacts, low spatial resolution, and low signal-to-noise ratio.[1]

Contrast-enhanced MR pulmonary perfusion
Dynamic time-resolved MR sequence is obtained with subtracted first-pass dynamic postcontrast T1-weighted imaging with high temporal resolution. A lower quantity of gadolinium contrast such as 0.05 to 0.1 mmol/kg is used.[6] Perfusion imaging has higher temporal but lower spatial

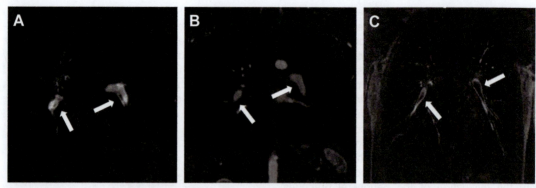

Fig. 1. Examples of Maki artifact. (*A*) Coronal high-resolution 3D T1-weighted MRA image shows central filling defects in bilateral pulmonary artery branches. (*B*) A delayed-phase MRA image from the same patient shows resolution of the filling defects. Findings are consistent with Maki artifact. Obtaining a delayed phase imaging is essential in distinguishing the artifact from thrombus. (*C*) Coronal MRA image shows Maki artifact mimicking a pulmonary embolism in another patient.

resolution than MR angiography. The perfusion images could be obtained with breath holds or free breathing.[11] A 3D FLASH MR imaging is frequently employed.[18] The perfusion abnormalities identified with this technique can be qualitatively and quantitatively assessed.[11]

Although the perfusion MR imaging technique has been studied for more than 20 years and significant advancements have been made, the clinical translation of these improvements has been relatively slow. This is primarily due to high feasibility of other studies such as single-photon emission computed tomography (SPECT) and spectral CT.[6] However, MR imaging may have a potential role in pregnant and pediatric patients and patients requiring serial imaging.[19] Dynamic contrast-enhanced lung perfusion MR imaging has similar sensitivity and specificity to SPECT and planar scintigraphy for screening for chronic thromboembolic pulmonary hypertension.[20,21]

IMAGING PROTOCOL

In our institution, MR pulmonary angiography examinations are performed using at least 1.5 T field magnetic strength. The chest imaging begins with axial and coronal 2 dimensional (2D) bSSFP and axial and coronal fat-saturated T1-weighted spoiled gradient echo sequences. Subsequently, an initial mask of a high-resolution (HR) 3D T1 gradient echo data set is acquired during breath hold at end expiration. Before contrast administration, the technologists check the images for wrap-around artifacts and coach the patient on breath-hold instructions. A single dose of gadolinium-based contrast (0.1 mmol/kg) is prepared and diluted with saline at a 1:1 ratio. Coronal TR-MRA is acquired with a temporal resolution of 2 seconds, which begins immediately before the contrast injection. Initially, 5 to 8 mL of the diluted contrast (~25%–30% of the total contrast amount) is administered at a rate of 2 mL/sec. Subsequently, the remainder of the contrast is injected at a rate of 2 mL/sec, and the coronal HR MRA images are acquired, which is timed to pulmonary arteries. After HR MRA images, a coronal whole-heart 3D Nav inversion revocery (IR) cardiac-gated and respiratory-gated images are obtained. Then, postcontrast axial and coronal fat-saturated T1-weighted spoiled gradient echo sequences are acquired (**Table 1**). Total table time is 30 to 45 minutes. Post-processing is performed at the scanner, which includes maximum intensity project images and axial-plane multiplanar reformation of the HR-MRA, 3D Nav-IR MRA, and TR-MRA (during the maximum opacification of the pulmonary artery) and images are sent to picture archiving and communication system. It is possible to create a significantly abbreviated protocol to allow for more rapid evaluation for acute pulmonary embolism. In this setting, an HR-MRA can be timed to the pulmonary artery phase of enhancement, followed by 2 to 3 additional delayed-phased HR-MRA acquisitions (**Table 2**).[22]

IMAGING FINDINGS IN PULMONARY EMBOLISM

The imaging findings of pulmonary embolism with MRA are similar to those observed with CTA. Direct findings include filling defects, T1 hyperintense clot in the pulmonary arteries, occlusion of the pulmonary artery, and arterial cut-off sign (**Figs. 2**A–E and **3**A–C). Indirect signs include main pulmonary artery enlargement, dilated right heart chambers,

Table 1
Our institutional protocol

Preliminary Imaging	Three-plane Localizer Scout Imaging
Precontrast Sequences in Order	Axial bSSFP single-shot, breath hold Coronal bSSFP single-shot, breath hold Axial fat-saturated T1W spoiled GRE, breath hold Coronal fat-saturated T1W spoiled GRE, breath hold Coronal high-resolution precontrast 3D T1W GRE MRA, breath hold
Contrast Agent Injection	Intravenous single dose of gadolinium-based contrast 0.1 mmol/kg which is diluted with saline at 1:1 ratio
Postcontrast Sequences in Order	Coronal time-resolved MRA (temporal resolution of 2 s), 5–8 mL bolus at 2 mL/sec rate, scan starts immediately prior to injection Coronal high-resolution 3D T1W GRE MRA, breath hold, injection of the remainder of contrast at 2 mL/sec, timed to pulmonary artery Coronal whole heart 3D Navigator IR cardiac and respiratory gated Axial fat-saturated T1W spoiled GRE, breath hold Coronal fat-saturated T1W spoiled GRE, breath hold

peripheral wedge-shaped intensities representing pulmonary infarcts, pleural effusion, atelectasis, and perfusion defects on MR imaging perfusion.[1,17]

CLINICAL APPLICATIONS
Acute Pulmonary Embolism

CT pulmonary angiography is the reference standard first-line imaging tool for assessing pulmonary embolism.[4] Historically, due to its limitations, MRA has not been a preferred diagnostic test. In 2010, Prospective Investigation of Pulmonary Embolism Diagnosis III efficacy study revealed that contrast-enhanced MR angiography is technically insufficient in 25% of the patients. Technically adequate studies had a high specificity (99%) and a moderate sensitivity (78%). The success of pulmonary embolism detection has gradually decreased in peripheral pulmonary arteries; the sensitivity of detection of a subsegmental pulmonary embolism was 0%. The authors concluded that MR pulmonary angiography should be performed at institutions with experience and in cases where the other studies are contraindicated.[23] More recently, Repplinger and colleagues[24] demonstrated that in 1173 patients, 6 month major adverse pulmonary embolism-related events were higher in the CTA group compared to the MRA group. The technically adequate studies were comparable between CTA and MRA groups (90.5% vs 92.6%). Schiebler and colleagues[25] showed that 97.4% of the MR pulmonary angiography studies in their cohort were of diagnostic quality. Currently, per the American College of Radiology (ACR) appropriateness criteria for assessment of acute chest pain, the rating of MRA is 2 out of 10, and the rating of CTA is 5

Table 2
Abbreviated protocol of pulmonary MR angiography[22]

Preliminary Imaging	Three-Plane Localizer Scout Imaging
Precontrast Sequence	Coronal precontrast 3D T1W spoiled GRE MRA, breath hold
Contrast Agent Injection	Intravenous single dose of gadolinium-based contrast that is diluted with saline to a total volume of 30 mL and injected at 1.5 mL/s rate
Postcontrast Sequences in Order	Coronal 3D T1W spoiled GRE MRA, breath hold, timed to pulmonary artery Coronal 3D T1W spoiled GRE MRA, breath hold, immediate delay Low flip angle T1W 3D spoiled GRE MRA T1W 2D axial or 3D spoiled GRE with fat saturation

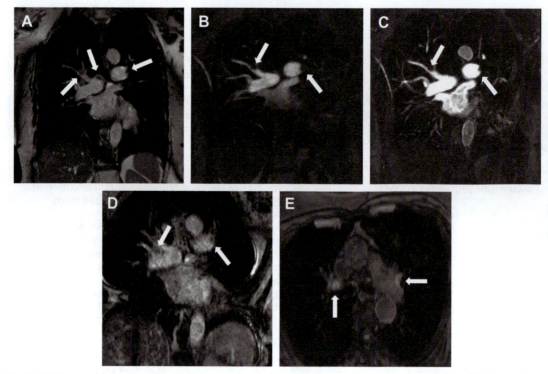

Fig. 2. A 70 year old woman with chest pain and prior history of severe iodine contrast allergy. (*A*) Coronal precontrast bSSFP, (*B*) coronal time-resolved MRA, (*C*) high-resolution 3D T1-weighted MRA, (*D*) navigator-gated 3D SSFP images demonstrate multifocal eccentric partial filling defects in the distal right, right upper lobe, and left interlobar pulmonary arteries representing chronic pulmonary embolism. (*E*) Axial precontrast T1-weighted GRE image demonstrates intrinsic T1 hyperintense signal of the thrombus.

out of 10 in intermediate probability with a negative D-dimer or in low pretest probability. The rating of the MRA is 6 out of 10, and the CTA is 9 out of 10 in intermediate probability with a positive D-dimer or in high pretest probability.[26] Relatively recent meta-analyses showed that MRA was a better diagnostic tool than CTA for detecting pulmonary embolism.[27,28] A meta-analysis in 2023 demonstrated that MRA showed the best diagnostic performance for diagnosing pulmonary embolism with a sensitivity of 93% and specificity of 94%.[28] Starekova and colleagues[5] demonstrated that the

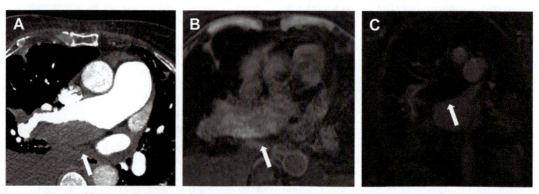

Fig. 3. A 73 year old woman with history of hepatocellular carcinoma. (*A*) Axial CT image demonstrates a partially occlusive eccentric hypodense filling defect that is suspicious for tumor or bland thrombus. (*B*) Axial precontrast T1-weighted GRE image demonstrates intrinsic T1 hyperintense signal within the abnormality. (*C*) Coronal subtraction postcontrast T1-weighted image demonstrates no definitive contrast enhancement within the abnormality. Findings are suggestive of bland thrombus rather than tumor thrombus given no definitive enhancement of the lesion and intrinsic T1 hyperintensity.

use of pulmonary MRA instead of CTA for the assessment of pulmonary embolism aided to preserve iodinated contrast media during the contrast media shortage in 2022, and MRA could be a feasible alternative to CTA for pulmonary embolism evaluation in emergency settings.

Chronic Pulmonary Thromboembolic Disease

Chronic pulmonary thromboembolic disease (CTED) and chronic pulmonary thromboembolic pulmonary hypertension (CTEPH) are rare long-term complications of acute pulmonary embolism with organized clot obstructing the pulmonary arteries. Diagnostic assessment includes echocardiography, ventilation-perfusion (V/Q) scanning, CT pulmonary angiography, right heart catheterization, and catheter pulmonary angiography.[29] MR pulmonary angiography and perfusion MR imaging may be feasible for assessing CTED and CTEPH. Johns and colleagues[21] showed that perfusion MR imaging has a higher sensitivity (100%) in diagnosing CTEPH and CTED when compared to SPECT (97%) with a similar specificity (81%). Furthermore, cardiac MR imaging with cine imaging provides a complete functional and morphologic assessment of the right ventricular size and function.[29] Deux and colleagues[30] demonstrated that vortex duration in the main pulmonary artery on 4 dimensional (4D) flow may noninvasively detect pulmonary hypertension. Cardiac MR imaging and perfusion MR imaging are emerging tools for monitoring during treatment or after surgery. Czerner and colleagues[31] showed that pulmonary hemodynamics obtained by 2D phase contrast images accurately reflect the pulmonary blood flow changes in patients with CTEPH after endarterectomy. Ohno and colleagues[32] demonstrated that dynamic perfusion MR imaging could be used to monitor treatment effects in medically treated patients with CTEPH.

Pulmonary Hypertension

Pulmonary hypertension is progressive elevation of pulmonary artery pressure and is defined as mean pulmonary artery pressure greater than 20 mm Hg and pulmonary vascular resistance greater than 2.0 Wood units.[33] The classification of pulmonary hypertension consists of a heterogeneous group of diseases. Diagnostic evaluation includes echocardiography, V/Q scintigraphy, chest CT, cardiac MR imaging, and right heart catheterization.[34] Cardiac MR imaging is vital in establishing diagnosis, determining underlying etiology, and assessing the prognosis and therapy response.[7] Furthermore, quantitative perfusion MR imaging may have value in the assessment of pulmonary hypertension.[18]

Morphologic and functional analysis

Cine images obtained with bright-blood balanced-SSFP sequences with parallel short-axis images covering the heart provide information regarding right ventricle (RV) morphology and function. Cardiac MR imaging enables the most accurate and reproducible method of determination of RV volume, mass, and function.[7,35] A meta-analysis has shown that MR imaging may have a surrogate role as a noninvasive imaging technique to diagnose pulmonary hypertension and has higher sensitivity (92%) and specificity (86%) than echocardiography and CT (Fig. 4A, B, Videos 1 and 2).[36] The ventricular mass index can be calculated by the RV mass ratio to the left ventricle (LV) mass. A ventricular mass index greater than 0.45 can diagnose pulmonary hypertension with a sensitivity of 84% and specificity of 82%.[37] Johns and colleagues[38] showed that the combined use of interventricular septum angle, ventricular mass index, and slow flow at the black-blood imaging in the pulmonary artery can determine pulmonary hypertension with a sensitivity of 93% and specificity of 79%.

Cardiac MR imaging is a powerful tool to assess prognosis and treatment response. A meta-analysis showed that the most important prognostic factor was a decreased right ventricle ejection fraction (RVEF).[39] Lewis and colleagues[40] revealed that RVEF of less than 37% has a high risk of 1 year mortality. Furthermore, increase in RV end-diastolic and end-systolic volumes and decrease in LV end-diastolic and LV stroke volumes are associated with increased mortality.[41] Johns and colleagues[42] demonstrated that an interventricular septal angle greater than 160° can identify patients with combined precapillary and postcapillary pulmonary hypertension and predict those at risk for a poor outcome.

Furthermore, cardiac MR imaging can provide additional structural and functional information, including determination of the concentric or eccentric hypertrophy, presence of interventricular coupling, size of the pulmonary artery, and right atrial enlargement.[7] Strain analysis with cardiac MR imaging is beneficial in for determining severity and risk assessment of pulmonary hypertension.[7]

Hemodynamic analysis

Pulmonary hypertension is characterized by increased pulmonary vascular resistance, decreased cardiac output, and altered pulmonary blood flow. Slow flow may be detected with black-blood imaging technique or phase contrast

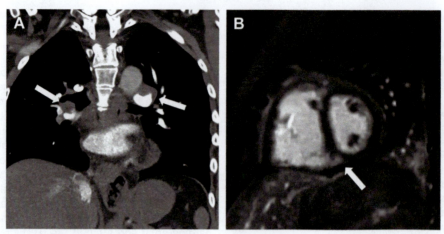

Fig. 4. A 45 year old woman with chronic pulmonary thromboembolism. (*A*) Coronal chest CT image demonstrates eccentric thrombi in bilateral interlobar pulmonary arteries. (*B*) Short-axis late gadolinium enhancement image demonstrates midmyocardial delayed enhancement in the mid-inferior right ventricle insertion point.

imaging.[43] Black-blood MR imaging is acquired with a gated spin-echo double inversion recovery sequence, which nulls the signal from the fast-flowing blood. In pulmonary hypertension, slow or turbulent flow appears as a smoky intermediate signal within the vessel lumen.[7,43] Prolonged RV-to-LV pulmonary transit time on first-pass dynamic contrast imaging may occur in patients with pulmonary hypertension.[44]

Phase contrast imaging is used for quantitative hemodynamic assessment of the pulmonary arteries. 2D phase contrast imaging is acquired throughout the cardiac cycle with gradient echo imaging perpendicular to the main pulmonary artery with velocity encoding direction along the pulmonary artery flow. Usually, a velocity encoding value of 150 cm/s is used to assess the pulmonary artery. With 2D phase contrast imaging, pulmonary artery dimensions, velocities, and stiffness could be assessed.[7,43] A cut-off pulmonary artery average velocity value of 11.7 cm/s may diagnose pulmonary hypertension with a sensitivity of 92.9% and specificity of 82.4%.[45] Ray and colleagues demonstrated that the percent change of pulmonary artery cross-sectional area during the cardiac cycle of less than 40% could determine pulmonary hypertension with a sensitivity of 95% and specificity of 94%. The area change could reflect the disease severity and prognosis.[46,47] Arterial stiffness could also be assessed with pulse wave velocity (PWV), which may have a diagnostic and prognostic value. PWV information could be obtained with phase contrast images at the main, right, and left pulmonary arteries. PWV is calculated with the distance between the sampled regions and the temporal delay between the waveforms.[7,43]

The 4D phase-contrast technique (4D flow) allows for volumetric time-resolved 3D velocity-encoding imaging. It enables comprehensive analysis of complex blood flow overtime. Slow flow and abnormal flow patterns have been demonstrated in patients with pulmonary hypertension. Furthermore, 4D flow imaging could be used for the evaluation of flow through the tricuspid valve.[7]

Tissue characterization

Areas of myocardial scarring or fibrosis can be assessed with late gadolinium enhancement (LGE) imaging. The LGE sequences are obtained approximately 10 minutes after administration of the gadolinium-based contrast with gradient echo imaging using a 180° inversion. In patients with pulmonary hypertension, the typical pattern is mid-myocardial LGE in the RV insertion points sometimes involving the interventricular septum (see **Fig. 4**). The distribution of LGE is likely related to strain onto the interventricular septum due to increased RV pressures and RV dysfunction.[7,43]

T1 mapping and extracellular volume (ECV) calculation enable quantification of the myocardial characteristics to evaluate alterations in myocardial composition.[48] Elevated native T1 and ECV values at the RV insertion points were reported in the setting of pulmonary hypertension.[7,43,49]

Pulmonary Artery Masses

Pulmonary artery sarcoma (PAS) is rare and highly aggressive neoplasm with poor prognosis. It usually involves the central pulmonary arteries. The diagnosis of PAS can be challenging as the clinical presentation and CT imaging findings can mimic acute or chronic pulmonary embolism. MR

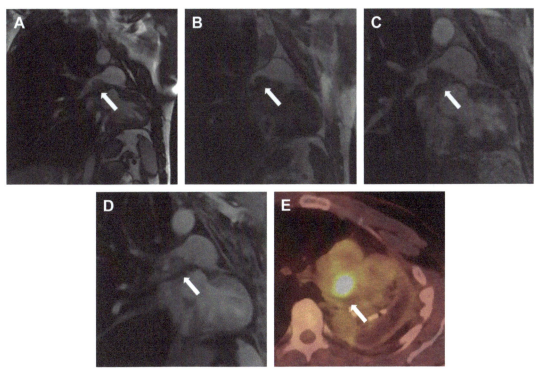

Fig. 5. A 49 year old man with a history of pulmonary artery sarcoma treated with left pneumectomy. On surveillance follow-up MR imaging, (A) coronal SSFP and (B) coronal time-resolved MRA image show a partially occlusive lobulated heterogenous lesion in the right pulmonary artery. (C) Coronal high-resolution 3D T1-weighted MRA and (D) coronal postcontrast T1-weighted GRE image demonstrate heterogenous enhancement of the mass. (E) Axial FDG-PET/CT image shows abnormal FDG-avid activity in the lesion. Findings are consistent with recurrence of the sarcoma with tumor thrombus in the right pulmonary artery.

imaging may provide additional information in characterization and differentiation.[50] With increased soft tissue characterization, ECG-gated cardiac MR imaging could better delineate the relationship between the tumor and surrounding structures and assess the intravascular or extravascular extension. The MR imaging signal of the sarcoma is highly variable on T1-weighted and T2-weighted images.

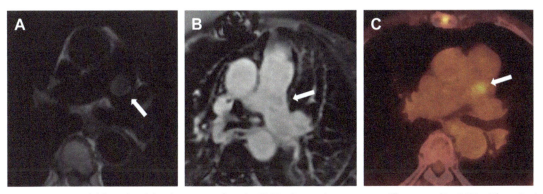

Fig. 6. A 69 year old female with a heart trasplant in 2017 who underwent surveillance cardiac MRI with an incidental pulmonary artery lesion. (A) The lesion demonstrates T2 hyperintensity. (B) Four chamber LGE images obtained with a long inversion time demonstrates enhancement of the lesion without associated low signal, compatible with an enhancing mass and not a thrombus. (C) Axial FDG-PET/CT image shows abnormal FDG-avid activity of the lesion. The lesion was resected, and the pathologic evaluation showed a benign lesion as a PIK3CA-mutated vascular overgrowth.

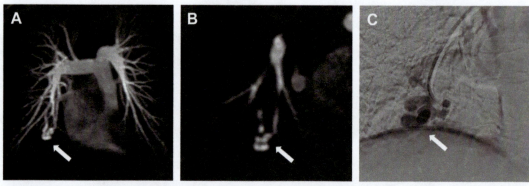

Fig. 7. A 72 year old woman with pulmonary arteriovenous malformation (AVM) in the right lower lobe. (*A*) and (*B*) Coronal time-resolved MRA images demonstrate abnormally dilated vessels representing an arteriovenous malformation with a single feeding segmental pulmonary artery branch. The AVM drains into a pulmonary vein. (*C*) Catheter angiography image confirms the diagnosis. The patient was treated with embolization.

Obtaining fat-suppressed T2-weighted mages can accentuate the T2 signal of the lesion. The most helpful sequences in distinguishing neoplasm from thrombus are postcontrast imaging (see **Fig. 3**; **Figs. 5**A–E and **6**A–C and Videos 3–5). Obtaining dynamic postcontrast images or multiphasic sequences with arterial and delayed phases may demonstrate tumor enhancement. Post-processing with subtraction imaging is helpful as it accentuates enhancement. However, the degree of enhancement varies in PAS, and the absence of enhancement does not exclude the diagnosis.[51,52]

Vasculitis

Takayasu arteritis and giant cell arteritis (GCA) usually involve the aorta and its larger branches; however, the pulmonary arteries may also be affected.[3] MR imaging findings of GCA and Takayasu arteritis are similar and include thickening of the affected pulmonary artery wall during the acute phase. Obtaining a delayed phase postcontrast imaging may delineate wall enhancement, which indicates inflammation. Occlusion and pseudoaneurysm formation may also be detected during the acute phase. MR imaging

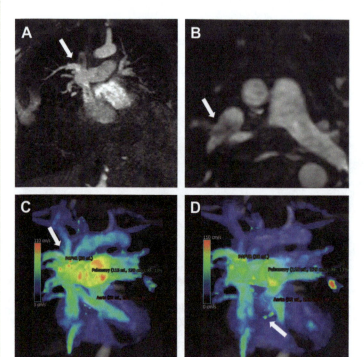

Fig. 8. A 69 year old man with shortness of breath and dilated right ventricle reported on echocardiography. (*A*) Maximum intensity project (MIP) coronal time-resolved MRA and (*B*) axial multiplanar reformation (MPR) navigator-gated 3D SSFP images demonstrate right upper lobe pulmonary vein draining into the superior vena cava, representing a partial anomalous pulmonary venous return (PAPVR). (*C*) Four dimensional (4D) flow demonstrates the PAPVR. Pulmonary-systemic flow (Qp/Qs) ratio is calculated as 1.4. (*D*) Additionally, with 4D flow imaging, a small incidental atrial septal defect is noted.

findings during the chronic phase include pulmonary artery stenosis and occlusions.[53] Behçet disease involves both arteries and veins and is the most common cause of pulmonary artery aneurysm. Additionally, thrombosis, aneurysms, and occlusions of the pulmonary artery branches may occur.[54] The main limitation of the MRA is the poor delineation of the distal pulmonary artery branches. However, MR imaging could be beneficial for surveillance imaging without additional ionizing radiation exposure.[53]

Additional Uses of Cardiovascular MR Imaging in Congenital and Acquired Pulmonary Vascular Diseases

MR pulmonary angiography is helpful in the structural evaluation of congenital and acquired pulmonary artery diseases, including aneurysms, stenosis, atresia, anomalous origin of pulmonary artery, and shunts such as arteriovenous malformations and patent ductus arteriosus (Fig. 7A–C).[3,11] Furthermore, functional assessment with 2D or 4D phase contrast imaging provides quantification of the flows and shunt volumes. Acquisition of same-session dedicated cardiac imaging sequences may allow a complete assessment of the cardiovascular morphology and function.[55]

MR pulmonary venography enables assessing pulmonary venous anatomy and diseases.[11] TR-MRA of pulmonary veins provides diagnostic quality images in pulmonary vein assessment for preprocedural planning for radiofrequency ablation in atrial fibrillation.[14] Furthermore, MR pulmonary venography aids the diagnosis of pulmonary venous diseases such as anomalous pulmonary venous return, pulmonary vein stenosis, and hypoplasia/atresia (Fig. 8A–D).[56]

SUMMARY

Cardiac MR imaging and pulmonary MRA are important clinical tools for the assessment of pulmonary vascular diseases. There are evolving non-contrast and contrast-enhanced techniques to evaluate pulmonary vasculature. Pulmonary MR angiography is a feasible imaging alternative to CTA in pulmonary embolism detection. Perfusion MR imaging and cardiac MR imaging help diagnose and monitor the treatment response of chronic thromboembolic pulmonary hypertension. Cardiac MR imaging is pivotal in assessing the potential underlying etiology and impact of pulmonary hypertension on the heart by providing reference-standard noninvasive cardiac morphology and function assessment and tissue characterization. Multiphasic acquisitions and dynamic phase imaging are unique to pulmonary MRA, which aid in diagnosing many pulmonary vascular diseases, including shunts and masses.

CLINICS CARE POINTS

- Cardiac MR imaging and pulmonary MRA are important imaging tools to assess pulmonary vascular diseases.
- Pulmonary MR angiography is a feasible imaging alternative to CTA in pulmonary embolism detection.
- Perfusion MR imaging and cardiac MR imaging help diagnose and monitor the treatment response of chronic thromboembolic pulmonary hypertension.
- Cardiac MR imaging is pivotal in assessing the potential underlying etiology and impact of pulmonary hypertension on the heart by providing reference-standard noninvasive cardiac morphology and function assessment and tissue characterization.
- Multiphasic acquisitions and dynamic phase imaging are unique to pulmonary MRA, which aid in diagnosing many pulmonary vascular diseases, including shunts and masses.

DISCLOSURE

The authors have nothing to disclose.

FUNDING

Dr Agirlar Trabonzlu has nothing to disclose. Dr Allen has the following disclosures: Co-Founder and Shareholder: Third Coast Dynamics, Inc.; Honoraria: Siemens, MRI Online, Circle Cardiovascular Imaging; Grant Support: Guerbet, NIH/NHLBI R01HL168700; Travel: Siemens; Expert Witness: Burns White.

SUPPLEMENTARY DATA

Supplementary data to this article can be found online at https://doi.org/10.1016/j.rcl.2024.09.003.

REFERENCES

1. Tsuchiya N, van Beek E Jr, Ohno Y, et al. Magnetic resonance angiography for the primary diagnosis of pulmonary embolism: a review from the international workshop for pulmonary functional imaging. World J Radiol 2018;10(6):52–64.
2. Ohno Y, Yoshikawa T, Kishida Y, et al. Unenhanced and contrast-enhanced MR angiography and perfusion

imaging for suspected pulmonary thromboembolism. AJR Am J Roentgenol 2017;208(3):517–30.
3. Leitman EM, McDermott S. Pulmonary arteries: imaging of pulmonary embolism and beyond. Cardiovasc Diagn Ther 2019;9(Suppl 1):S37–58.
4. Ley S, Kauczor HU. MR imaging/magnetic resonance angiography of the pulmonary arteries and pulmonary thromboembolic disease. Magn Reson Imaging Clin N Am 2008;16(2):263–273, ix.
5. Starekova J, Chu SY, Bluemke DA, et al. MRA as the preferred test for pulmonary embolism during the iodinated contrast media shortage of 2022: a single-center experience. AJR Am J Roentgenol 2023;221(6):736–46.
6. Kay FU, Madhuranthakam AJ. MR perfusion imaging of the lung. Magn Reson Imaging Clin N Am 2024;32(1):111–23.
7. Broncano J, Bhalla S, Gutierrez FR, et al. Cardiac MRI in pulmonary hypertension: from magnet to bedside. Radiographics 2020;40(4):982–1002.
8. Herédia V, Altun E, Ramalho M, et al. MRI of pregnant patients for suspected pulmonary embolism: steady-state free precession vs postgadolinium 3D-GRE. Acta Med Port 2012;25(6):359–67.
9. Kaya F, Ufuk F, Karabulut N. Diagnostic performance of contrast-enhanced and unenhanced combined pulmonary artery MRI and magnetic resonance venography techniques in the diagnosis of venous thromboembolism. Br J Radiol 2019;92(1095):20180695.
10. Hui BK, Noga ML, Gan KD, et al. Navigator-gated three-dimensional MR angiography of the pulmonary arteries using steady-state free precession. J Magn Reson Imaging 2005;21(6):831–5.
11. Aziz M, Krishnam M, Madhuranthakam AJ, et al. Update on MR imaging of the pulmonary vasculature. Int J Cardiovasc Imaging 2019;35(8):1483–97.
12. Hecht EM, Rosenkrantz A. Pulmonary MR angiography techniques and applications. Magn Reson Imaging Clin N Am 2009;17(1):101–31.
13. Cornfeld D, Mojibian H. Clinical uses of time-resolved imaging in the body and peripheral vascular system. AJR Am J Roentgenol 2009;193(6):W546–57.
14. Schonberger M, Usman A, Galizia M, et al. Time-resolved MR venography of the pulmonary veins precatheter-based ablation for atrial fibrillation. J Magn Reson Imaging 2013;37(1):127–37.
15. Bannas P, Schiebler ML, Motosugi U, et al. Pulmonary MRA: differentiation of pulmonary embolism from truncation artefact. Eur Radiol 2014;24(8):1942–9.
16. Starekova J, Nagle SK, Schiebler ML, et al. Pulmonary MRA during pregnancy: early experience with ferumoxytol. J Magn Reson Imaging 2023;57(6):1815–8.
17. Bergmann LL, Ackman JB, Starekova J, et al. MR angiography of pulmonary vasculature. Magn Reson Imaging Clin N Am 2023;31(3):475–91.
18. Lacharie M, Villa A, Milidonis X, et al. Role of pulmonary perfusion magnetic resonance imaging for the diagnosis of pulmonary hypertension: a review. World J Radiol 2023;15(9):256–73.
19. Hatabu H, Ohno Y, Gefter WB, et al. Expanding applications of pulmonary MRI in the clinical evaluation of lung disorders: fleischner society position paper. Radiology 2020;297(2):286–301.
20. Rajaram S, Swift AJ, Telfer A, et al. 3D contrast-enhanced lung perfusion MRI is an effective screening tool for chronic thromboembolic pulmonary hypertension: results from the ASPIRE Registry. Thorax 2013;68(7):677–8.
21. Johns CS, Swift AJ, Rajaram S, et al. Lung perfusion: MRI vs. SPECT for screening in suspected chronic thromboembolic pulmonary hypertension. J Magn Reson Imaging 2017;46(6):1693–7.
22. Benson DG, Schiebler ML, Repplinger MD, et al. Contrast-enhanced pulmonary MRA for the primary diagnosis of pulmonary embolism: current state of the art and future directions. Br J Radiol 2017;90(1074):20160901.
23. Stein PD, Chenevert TL, Fowler SE, et al. Gadolinium-enhanced magnetic resonance angiography for pulmonary embolism: a multicenter prospective study (PIOPED III). Ann Intern Med 2010;152(7):434–43. W142-3.
24. Repplinger MD, Nagle SK, Harringa JB, et al. Clinical outcomes after magnetic resonance angiography (MRA) versus computed tomographic angiography (CTA) for pulmonary embolism evaluation. Emerg Radiol 2018;25(5):469–77.
25. Schiebler ML, Nagle SK, François CJ, et al. Effectiveness of MR angiography for the primary diagnosis of acute pulmonary embolism: clinical outcomes at 3 months and 1 year. J Magn Reson Imaging 2013;38(4):914–25.
26. Kirsch J, Brown RKJ, Henry TS, et al, Expert Panels on Cardiac and Thoracic Imaging. ACR appropriateness Criteria® acute chest pain-suspected pulmonary embolism. J Am Coll Radiol 2017;14(5S):S2–12.
27. Chen F, Shen YH, Zhu XQ, et al. Comparison between CT and MRI in the assessment of pulmonary embolism: a meta-analysis. Medicine 2017;96(52):e8935.
28. Pagkalidou E, Doundoulakis I, Apostolidou-Kiouti F, et al. An overview of systematic reviews on imaging tests for diagnosis of pulmonary embolism applying different network meta-analytic methods. Hellenic J Cardiol 2024;76:88–98.
29. Hahn LD, Papamatheakis DG, Fernandes TM, et al. Multidisciplinary approach to chronic thromboembolic pulmonary hypertension: role of radiologists. Radiographics 2023;43(2):e220078.
30. Deux JF, Crowe LA, Genecand L, et al. Correlation between pulmonary artery pressure and vortex duration determined by 4D flow MRI in main

30. pulmonary artery in patients with suspicion of chronic thromboembolic pulmonary hypertension (CTEPH). J Clin Med Res 2022;11(17). https://doi.org/10.3390/jcm11175237.
31. Czerner CP, Schoenfeld C, Cebotari S, et al. Perioperative CTEPH patient monitoring with 2D phase-contrast MRI reflects clinical, cardiac and pulmonary perfusion changes after pulmonary endarterectomy. PLoS One 2020;15(9):e0238171.
32. Ohno Y, Koyama H, Yoshikawa T, et al. Contrast-enhanced multidetector-row computed tomography vs. Time-resolved magnetic resonance angiography vs. contrast-enhanced perfusion MRI: assessment of treatment response by patients with inoperable chronic thromboembolic pulmonary hypertension. J Magn Reson Imaging 2012;36(3):612–23.
33. Maron BA. Revised definition of pulmonary hypertension and approach to management: a clinical primer. J Am Heart Assoc 2023;12(8):e029024.
34. Crisan S, Baghina RM, Luca SA, et al. Comprehensive imaging in patients with suspected pulmonary arterial hypertension. Heart 2024;110(4):228–34.
35. Hulten EA, Bradley AJ. Cardiac magnetic resonance evaluation of pulmonary arterial hypertension: transforming from supplementary to primary imaging modality? JACC Cardiovasc Imaging 2021;14(5):943–6.
36. Ullah W, Minalyan A, Saleem S, et al. Comparative accuracy of non-invasive imaging versus right heart catheterization for the diagnosis of pulmonary hypertension: a systematic review and meta-analysis. Int J Cardiol Heart Vasc 2020;29:100568.
37. Wang N, Hu X, Liu C, et al. A systematic review of the diagnostic accuracy of cardiovascular magnetic resonance for pulmonary hypertension. Can J Cardiol 2014;30(4):455–63.
38. Johns CS, Kiely DG, Rajaram S, et al. Diagnosis of pulmonary hypertension with cardiac MRI: derivation and validation of regression models. Radiology 2019;290(1):61–8.
39. Dong Y, Pan Z, Wang D, et al. Prognostic value of cardiac magnetic resonance-derived right ventricular remodeling parameters in pulmonary hypertension: a systematic review and meta-analysis. Circ Cardiovasc Imaging 2020;13(7):e010568.
40. Lewis RA, Johns CS, Cogliano M, et al. Identification of cardiac magnetic resonance imaging thresholds for risk stratification in pulmonary arterial hypertension. Am J Respir Crit Care Med 2020;201(4):458–68.
41. Alabed S, Shahin Y, Garg P, et al. Cardiac-MRI predicts clinical worsening and mortality in pulmonary arterial hypertension: a systematic review and meta-analysis. JACC Cardiovasc Imaging 2021;14(5):931–42.
42. Johns CS, Wild JM, Rajaram S, et al. Identifying at-risk patients with combined pre- and postcapillary pulmonary hypertension using interventricular septal angle at cardiac MRI. Radiology 2018;289(1):61–8.
43. Saunders LC, Hughes PJC, Alabed S, et al. Integrated cardiopulmonary MRI assessment of pulmonary hypertension. J Magn Reson Imaging 2022;55(3):633–52.
44. Skrok J, Shehata ML, Mathai S, et al. Pulmonary arterial hypertension: MR imaging-derived first-pass bolus kinetic parameters are biomarkers for pulmonary hemodynamics, cardiac function, and ventricular remodeling. Radiology 2012;263(3):678–87.
45. Sanz J, Kuschnir P, Rius T, et al. Pulmonary arterial hypertension: noninvasive detection with phase-contrast MR imaging. Radiology 2007;243(1):70–9.
46. Swift AJ, Rajaram S, Condliffe R, et al. Pulmonary artery relative area change detects mild elevations in pulmonary vascular resistance and predicts adverse outcome in pulmonary hypertension. Invest Radiol 2012;47(10):571–7.
47. Ray JC, Burger C, Mergo P, et al. Pulmonary arterial stiffness assessed by cardiovascular magnetic resonance imaging is a predictor of mild pulmonary arterial hypertension. Int J Cardiovasc Imaging 2019;35(10):1881–92.
48. Hamlin SA, Henry TS, Little BP, et al. Mapping the future of cardiac MR imaging: case-based review of T1 and T2 mapping techniques. Radiographics 2014;34(6):1594–611.
49. García-Álvarez A, García-Lunar I, Pereda D, et al. Association of myocardial T1-mapping CMR with hemodynamics and RV performance in pulmonary hypertension. JACC Cardiovasc Imaging 2015;8(1):76–82.
50. Ropp AM, Burke AP, Kligerman SJ, et al. Intimal sarcoma of the great vessels. Radiographics 2021;41(2):361–79.
51. von Falck C, Meyer B, Fegbeutel C, et al. Imaging features of primary sarcomas of the great vessels in CT, MRI and PET/CT: a single-center experience. BMC Med Imaging 2013;13:25.
52. Liu M, Luo C, Wang Y, et al. Multiparametric MRI in differentiating pulmonary artery sarcoma and pulmonary thromboembolism: a preliminary experience. Diagn Interv Radiol 2017;23(1):15–21.
53. Sueyoshi E, Sakamoto I, Uetani M. MRI of takayasu's arteritis: typical appearances and complications. Am J Roentgenol 2006;187(6):W569–75.
54. Ceylan N, Bayraktaroglu S, Erturk SM, et al. Pulmonary and vascular manifestations of Behcet disease: imaging findings. AJR Am J Roentgenol 2010;194(2):W158–64.
55. Ntsinjana HN, Hughes ML, Taylor AM. The role of cardiovascular magnetic resonance in pediatric congenital heart disease. J Cardiovasc Magn Reson 2011;13(1):51.
56. Dillman JR, Yarram SG, Hernandez RJ. Imaging of pulmonary venous developmental anomalies. AJR Am J Roentgenol 2009;192(5):1272–85.

Pulmonary Vascular Interventions

Grace Laidlaw, MD, MS*, Hugh McGregor, MD, Karim Valji, MD

KEYWORDS

- Endovascular • Pulmonary • Thromboembolism • Malformation • Hemoptysis • Embolization

KEY POINTS

- Pulmonary vasculature is susceptible to a range of pathologies, including thromboembolic, inflammatory, infectious, neoplastic, traumatic, congenital/hereditary, and iatrogenic diseases.
- Minimally invasive endovascular techniques have largely supplanted surgical management of many pulmonary vascular diseases.
- A thorough understanding of the indications, contraindications, evidence for, and technical approaches to pulmonary vascular interventions is the key in ensuring safe, effective endovascular management of pulmonary vascular diseases.

INTRODUCTION

Critical functions of the lungs include gas exchange and blood filtration. These roles are facilitated by a network of pulmonary arteries and pulmonary veins, with bronchial arteries providing additional vascular supply to major airways. The presence of multiple vascular beds renders the lungs susceptible to diverse pathologies, including acute or chronic thromboembolic disease; infectious, inflammatory, or traumatic injuries; pulmonary arteriovenous malformations; and foreign body embolization. With improvements in endovascular techniques, endovascular management of these pathologies has either supplanted or plays an important complementary role to surgical interventions. This article reviews indications, contraindications, techniques, and outcomes in endovascular management of common pulmonary vascular pathologies, with the goal of improving operator familiarity and facility with these procedures.

PULMONARY DIGITAL SUBTRACTION ANGIOGRAPHY

Though more recently supplanted by computed tomography (CT), pulmonary digital subtraction angiography (DSA) has long been the gold standard for characterizing pulmonary artery (PA) anatomy and pathology and remains a critical diagnostic step in many PA interventions. Pulmonary DSA also plays an important role in preoperative planning for PA operations such as pulmonary endarterectomy. In some settings, the ability to measure PA pressures (PAP) is critical in guiding therapy.

Contraindications to pulmonary DSA are few. Pre-existing left bundle branch block is a relative contraindication, as right heart catheterization can induce transient right bundle branch block. The risk of complete heart block in these patients can be mitigated with temporary pacing systems that can be activated if needed. Patients may present with severe pulmonary hypertension (PH), precluding moderate sedation, but the procedure may be performed with minimal sedation or local anesthesia only. Pulmonary DSA is classified as low bleeding risk by the Society of Interventional Radiology (SIR), with a platelet threshold of greater than 20,000 and international normalized ratio (INR) less than 2.0 to 3.0.[1] The procedure can be done safely even with full anticoagulation, which should be continued in patients with history of thromboembolism.

Section of Interventional Radiology, Department of Radiology, University of Washington, Box 357233, 1959 Northeast Pacific Street, Seattle, WA 98195, USA
* Corresponding author.
E-mail address: gracel7@uw.edu

Pulmonary DSA begins with internal jugular (IJ) or common femoral vein (CFV) access in standard ultrasound-guided Seldinger fashion. After sheath placement, a flush catheter and wire are used to catheterize the main, right, or left PA (depending on procedural indication) under fluoroscopic guidance. PAP measurements can be obtained, followed by DSA.[2] Projections for angiography (biplane frontal and lateral, ipsilateral posterior oblique) and non-ionic contrast injection rates vary by clinical condition (Fig. 1A-F).[3,4]

Diagnostic pulmonary angiography is well-tolerated. Minor arrhythmias are common when traversing the right ventricle, but major arrhythmias requiring intervention are uncommon. Regardless, continuous cardiac monitoring and defibrillation equipment must be available. In 707 consecutive patients undergoing diagnostic pulmonary arteriography over 4 years, minor to moderate complication rates (including transient angina, access site hematoma, and urticaria) were 1.4%, with only 1 major reported complication (inadvertent femoral artery injury requiring operative repair).[3]

CATHETER-DIRECTED MANAGEMENT OF PULMONARY EMBOLISM

Acute pulmonary embolism (PE) is an important contributor to morbidity and mortality in the United States.[5] Acute PE can be stratified into massive, submassive, or low-risk categories depending on clinical variables, including the presence or absence of sustained hypotension, imaging or electrocardiography (EKG) evidence of right ventricular dysfunction, and biochemical evidence of myocardial strain.[6] Massive, submassive, and low-risk PEs have short-term mortality rates of 25% to 65%, 3% to 15%, and less than 1%, respectively, even if treated.[5]

Low-risk PE may be managed with therapeutic anticoagulation alone.[7] Massive PEs and, in some circumstances, submassive PEs require treatment to re-establish pulmonary perfusion and relieve right heart strain. Treatment has historically included therapeutic anticoagulation and/or systemic thrombolysis. Endovascular therapies that reduce or bypass thrombolytic administration, such as catheter-directed thrombolysis (CDT) or thrombectomy, have provided new tools in the treatment of massive and submassive PE.[8] Full review of the evidence supporting thrombectomy and CDT is beyond the scope of this article, but multiple studies have demonstrated promising improvements in hemodynamic parameters and imaging evidence of right heart strain, though adequately-powered, randomized trials are lacking.[9-18] Based on these results, catheter-based thrombectomy is recommended for massive PE

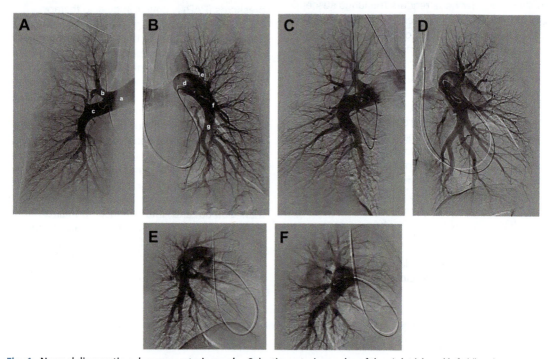

Fig. 1. Normal diagnostic pulmonary arteriography. Selective arteriography of the right (a) and left (d) pulmonary arteries in anteroposterior (A, B), 30° contralateral oblique (C, D), and lateral (E, F) views facilitates multiplanar vessel evaluation. The right pulmonary artery (PA) (a) divides into the truncus anterior (b), supplying anterior and apical segments of the right upper lobe. The interlobar pulmonary artery (c) gives rise to the upper lobe posterior segmental and multiple middle and lower lobe segmental arteries. The left PA (d) gives off upper lobe apicoposterior and anterior segmental arteries (e), and then gives rise to multiple lingular (f) and lower lobe (g) segmental arteries.

requiring immediate intervention before thrombolysis can take effect, after failed thrombolysis, or in patients with contraindications to thrombolysis.[7]

Contraindications to endovascular PE treatments vary by technique employed. Contraindications to CDT include active bleeding; recent major trauma, surgery, or intracranial injury; intracranial or spinal neoplasm; stroke within 6 months; and bleeding diatheses. Mechanical thrombectomy is more reasonable in these circumstances.[19] The SIR classifies PE interventions as high bleeding risk, with goal platelets greater than 50,000 and INR less than 1.5 to 1.8,[1] though anticoagulation should be continued if already initiated. As patients may present with tenuous hemodynamics and as catheter-based therapies may induce arrhythmias, endovascular PE interventions at the authors' institution are performed with anesthesiology assistance.

Catheter-based PE intervention begins with CFV access, favored over IJ access as this facilitates navigation of larger-bore thrombectomy devices. After placement of an appropriately-sized sheath, main PA catheterization, pressure measurements, and diagnostic angiography are performed as described in this article's first section. Intervention can then be pursued at the discretion of the treating interventionist.

If mechanical thrombectomy is pursued, the venous access sheath is upsized, and a coaxial thrombectomy device is advanced over a wire until the target embolus is reached (**Fig. 2**B and E). A bolus dose of therapeutic heparin (50–100 units/kg) is given during device insertion, as large-bore devices may otherwise induce thrombus. Available devices include manual vacuum catheters (FlowTriever Aspiration System, Inari Medical, Irvine, CA; AlphaVac, Angiodynamics, Latham, NY) or mechanized aspiration pumps (Lightning/Indigo Aspiration System, Penumbra Inc, Alameda, CA) (**Fig. 2**B and E). Multiple passes may be made with each device before removal. Pulmonary DSA and PAP measurements are performed following thrombectomy to confirm angiographic decrease in thrombus burden and/or reduction in PAP (**Fig. 2**C and F).

If catheter-directed thrombolysis is instead desired, single or dual infusion or flush catheters can be positioned central to or across the regions of embolus. Often, a bolus of tissue plasminogen activator (tPA) is given through each catheter, followed by tPA infusion via the lysis catheters and heparin infusion via the sheath sidearm. The patient returns for repeat arteriography within 24 hours, with catheter removal if thrombolysis is successful. If significant embolus burden remains, infusion catheters may be left in place for an additional 24 hours, though tPA infusions greater than 48 hours are not recommended. Enhanced catheter-directed thrombolysis devices, such as

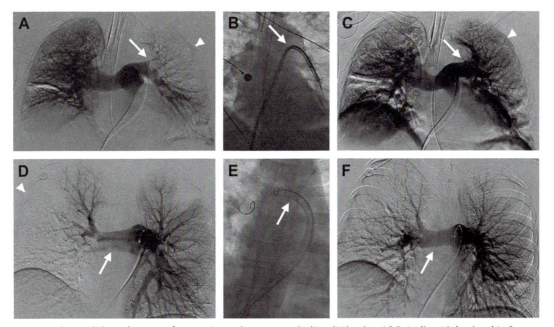

Fig. 2. Mechanical thrombectomy for massive pulmonary embolism (PE) using 16 Fr Indigo Lightning (*A–C, arrow in B*) (Penumbra) and 24 Fr FlowTriever (*D–F, arrow in E*) (Inari) devices. (*A* and *D*) Pulmonary arteriography demonstrates occlusive PE (*arrows*) and decreased pulmonary parenchymal perfusion (*arrowheads*). (*C* and *F*) After mechanical thrombectomy, there is no residual central embolism (*arrows*) and improved pulmonary parenchymal perfusion (*arrowhead*).

the EKOS ultrasonic CDT (USCDT) catheter (Boston Scientific, Marlborough, MA), which combines thrombolysis with high-frequency ultrasound, or the Bashir endovascular catheter (Thrombolex Inc, New Britain, PA), which combines pharmacologic thrombolysis with mechanical clot maceration, may alternatively be used.[20–22]

Catheter-based PE therapies are associated with low complication rates, though complications vary by treatment type. CDT and USCDT carry an increased risk of bleeding (1.8% and 5%, respectively) relative to therapeutic anticoagulation.[10,11] Major bleeding is less likely in patients undergoing mechanical thrombectomy, with reported rates of 0.9% to 1.6%.[15–17] However, large-bore mechanical thrombectomy devices predispose to other complications, including PA or cardiac injury or cardiovascular collapse (0.8%–1.0%); 30-day mortality estimates range from 0.8% to 1.0%.[15–17]

BALLOON PULMONARY ANGIOPLASTY FOR CHRONIC THROMBOEMBOLIC PULMONARY HYPERTENSION

Chronic thromboembolic pulmonary hypertension (CTEPH) arises when acute pulmonary thromboembolism evolves into chronic intravascular scar, leading to chronic precapillary pulmonary hypertension (PH) (mean PAP $\geq$25 mm Hg and PA wedge pressure $\leq$15 mm Hg).[23] While uncommon, with an incidence of 0.4% to 6.2% after pulmonary embolism, CTEPH is a source of prolonged morbidity after acute PE.[24] The diagnosis of CTEPH is imaging-driven; ventilation-perfusion scans show significantly mismatched perfusion, and pulmonary DSA and pulmonary arterial-phase chest CT demonstrate vessel irregularities, outpouchings, intraluminal webs, stenoses, or occlusions.[4]

While anticoagulation and medical management is critical in CTEPH care, pulmonary thromboendarterectomy (PEA) is the only definitive treatment. In patients with proximal thromboembolism and acceptable comorbidities, PEA is indicated.[25] However, balloon pulmonary angioplasty (BPA) is a promising alternative to surgery in select patients who are not operative candidates due to distal clot burden or severe comorbidities, or in those with residual PH after PEA. Multiple trials have shown that BPA improves 6-min walk distance, mean PAP, functional class, and quality of life in patients relative to medical management.[23,25–30] Management decisions are complex, and patients should be referred to a specialized CTEPH center for multidisciplinary evaluation.[4]

Contraindications to BPA include large, central thromboemboli, for which angioplasty is likely ineffective.[31,32] Patients with parenchymal fibrosis supplied by target vessels are unlikely to benefit from endovascular intervention.[32] BPA is considered a high-bleeding- risk procedure with goal platelets greater than 50,000 and INR less than 1.5 to 1.8, though anticoagulant medications should be continued intraprocedurally.[1,32,33] BPA should be performed with little to no sedation, as anesthetics can cause cardiovascular collapse in this population.[32,33]

BPA is performed under fluoroscopic guidance. Venous access and PA catheterization is performed as described earlier, with CFV access preferred for ease of operation.[32] Following systemic heparinization, target pulmonary branch arteries are reached via a sheath and coaxial guiding catheters, through which selective DSA can be performed (**Fig. 3**A).[32] Lesions should be targeted with the goal of treating the largest perfusional deficits, but morphology on DSA can further guide treatment.[32,33] Once a target vessel is

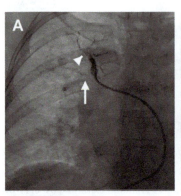
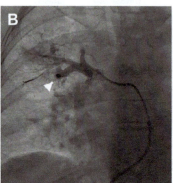
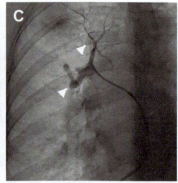

Fig. 3. Balloon pulmonary angioplasty (BPA) for chronic thromboembolic pulmonary hypertension (CTEPH). (A) Diagnostic pulmonary arteriography demonstrates chronic total occlusion (*arrow*) and irregularity (*arrowhead*) of right upper segmental pulmonary artery branches. (B, C) After balloon angioplasty, there is restored branch flow (*arrowheads*).

identified, a microwire is advanced across the lesion. Distal balloon angioplasty begins with small-diameter (often 2.0 mm), compliant balloons; proximal segments may be treated with sequentially larger balloons, though these should be smaller than the native target vessel diameter.[33,34] Treatment endpoints are based on improvements in regional pulmonary blood flow on pulmonary DSA and corresponding decreases in pressure (**Fig. 3**B and C).[35] Procedures may be repeated in multiple sessions, depending on the patient's reserve and anatomic complexity.[32,33]

While BPA outcomes were initially limited by reperfusion pulmonary edema in greater than 60% of patients, technical refinements have reduced complications, including wire injury, vessel dissection or rupture, parenchymal hemorrhage or hemothorax, hemoptysis, and pulmonary edema, to rates of less than 10% at experienced centers, with mortality rates of 3.9%.[31,36–38]

PULMONARY ARTERIOVENOUS MALFORMATION EMBOLIZATION

Pulmonary arteriovenous malformations (pAVMs) consist of abnormal direct connections between pulmonary arteries and pulmonary veins, creating right-to-left shunts. A total of 70% to 90% of individuals presenting with pAVMs have underlying hereditary hemorrhagic telangiectasia (HHT), though pAVMs may be sporadic or acquired secondary to trauma, cirrhosis, amyloidosis, or infection.[39,40]

Patients with pAVMs are often asymptomatic, though dyspnea and fatigue may be presenting symptoms. Symptom severity corresponds with pAVM size and degree of right-to-left shunting, which can affect oxygenation and result in paradoxic stroke, transient ischemic attack, and cerebral abscess.[39] Rationale for pAVM treatment even in asymptomatic patients is prevention of neurologic complications, other manifestations of paradoxic embolization, and (rarely) pulmonary hemorrhage.[40] While historical guidelines advocated for treatment of AVMs with feeding vessels larger than ≥ 3 mm, newer recommendations advocate for first-line endovascular intervention in all accessible pAVMs.[39,41,42] Resection or lung transplantation is reserved for rare cases of diffuse pAVM. Multiple observational studies have demonstrated high technical success rates, durable clinical success, and ischemic stroke rate reduction when state-of-the-art embolization techniques are employed.[39,42–48]

In addition to the contraindications to pulmonary DSA described at the beginning of this article, relative contraindications to pAVM treatment include complex or diffuse pAVMs not amenable to endovascular management.[47] pAVM embolization is considered a high- bleeding-risk procedure, with goal platelets greater than 50,000 and INR less than 1.5 to 1.8.[1]

pAVM embolization is performed under moderate sedation or general anesthesia, with the goal of facilitating breath-holds. Care should be taken to reduce paradoxical embolism and stroke risks, including use of intravenous line bubble filters, intraprocedural heparinization, catheter double-flushing, and removal of guidewires under saline baths. After PA catheterization, base and selective arteriography is performed in multiple projections to delineate the target pAVM (**Fig. 4**B and C). After feeding artery selection, embolization is performed using permanent embolic devices such as detachable coils or plugs. Embolization beginning within the sac or nidus is preferred over embolization of the feeding vessel alone[43,49–52] (**Fig. 4**D). Liquid or particle embolics should never be used, as these pose an unacceptable risk of paradoxic embolization. Post-embolization angiography is performed to ensure embolization of all feeding vessels (**Fig. 4**D). Multiple pAVMs may be treated in 1 session, though limiting treatment to a single lung is advocated by some practitioners. Following treatment, noncontrast or contrast-enhanced chest CT or bubble-study echocardiography may be used for surveillance.[39]

pAVM embolization is safe and well-tolerated. Major complication rates, including stroke, air embolism, PH exacerbation, pulmonary infarct, vessel injury, and access site complication, are 0.5% to 2%.[39,47] Pleuritic chest pain is the most common minor complication (15%–31%).[47] Post-treatment, up to 25% of patients may demonstrate pAVM reperfusion via recanalization or collateralized supply; re-treatment success rates are 40% to 80%.[39,44,53,54]

BRONCHIAL ARTERY EMBOLIZATION

Chronic pulmonary infection, inflammation, or malignancy can promote bronchial artery hypertrophy. Hypertrophied bronchial arteries are prone to hemorrhage, presenting as hemoptysis.[2] When bronchial artery hemorrhage results in greater than 300 mL of hemoptysis in 24 hours (defined as massive hemoptysis), mortality rates exceed 50% with conservative management.[55] In the absence of evidence of hemorrhage from the PA or other vascular beds, bronchial artery embolization (BAE) has become standard-of-care in massive hemoptysis, with surgery reserved for refractory cases.[55] BAE may also be reasonable in chronic hemoptysis refractory to medical

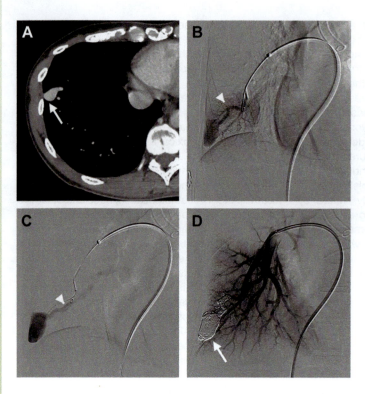

Fig. 4. Pulmonary arteriovenous malformations (pAVM) embolization. (A) Contrast-enhanced chest computed tomography (CT) reveals a right lower lobe pAVM (arrow). (B, C) Selective right lower pulmonary arteriography demonstrates a single feeding vessel (arrowhead, B) and draining vein (arrowhead, C). (D) After coil embolization of the nidus and feeding vessel, pulmonary arteriography demonstrates no residual filling of the pAVM (arrow).

management, as mortality rates of untreated nonmassive hemoptysis approach 5% to 21%.[56]

In the setting of hemoptysis, bronchoscopy may be used to localize bleeding, and chest CT may localize abnormal bronchial vessels or parasitized collaterals, show new parenchymal infiltrates that localize the region of bleeding, or exclude pseudoaneurysm or large vascular injury.[57] Active extravasation is rarely identified.[57] In life-threatening hemoptysis, the patient may be taken directly to angiography to minimize delays in care. While technically a low-bleeding-risk procedure, INR should be less than 1.8 if intervention is performed from a femoral approach, and less than 2.2 if a radial approach is used.[1] Intervention is often performed under general anesthesia; double-lumen intubation can be considered to isolate the unaffected lung.

Arterial access is obtained in standard fashion. Initial descending thoracic aortography is performed to identify culprit bronchial arteries, which have highly variable anatomy.[2] Selective bronchial arteriography is then performed, with typical findings including enlarged bronchial arteries, hypervascularity, and bronchial-pulmonary artery shunting (Fig. 5B and C). Frank extravasation is rare. When none of these findings are evident, systemic collateral arteries (eg, branches of subclavian, internal thoracic, intercostal, or inferior phrenic arteries) should be interrogated (Fig. 5D). Embolization is performed via a microcatheter advanced well into the target artery, avoiding reflux and nontarget embolization (Fig. 5E and F). Particle embolics are preferable, as these facilitate repeat embolization if hemoptysis recurs. BAE using coils or plugs is discouraged, as this hampers re-access in recurrent hemoptysis. Constant attention must be paid to filling of any vessels that could represent the anterior spinal artery (Fig. 5G). Inadvertent embolization of such branches may cause permanent paraplegia.

Despite this, BAE is a safe and effective technique for treating bronchial-origin hemoptysis, with technical success rates greater than 90% and immediate cessation of massive hemoptysis in 64% to 99% of patients.[55,57–60] Recurrent hemoptysis occurs in 9.8% to 57.5% of patients,[55,57,58] and nonbronchial systemic collaterals are associated with a higher rate of technical and clinical failure.[61] Chest pain is the most common minor complication, occurring in 5% to 9% of patients.[55,58] Major complications including nontarget embolization and access site complications occur in 0.0% to 6.6% of cases.[57]

INTERVENTIONS FOR PULMONARY ARTERIAL HEMORRHAGE

Fewer than 5% of hemoptysis episodes originate from the PA; these are usually infectious, traumatic, iatrogenic, postoperative, inflammatory, or malignant in etiology.[62] Patients undergoing

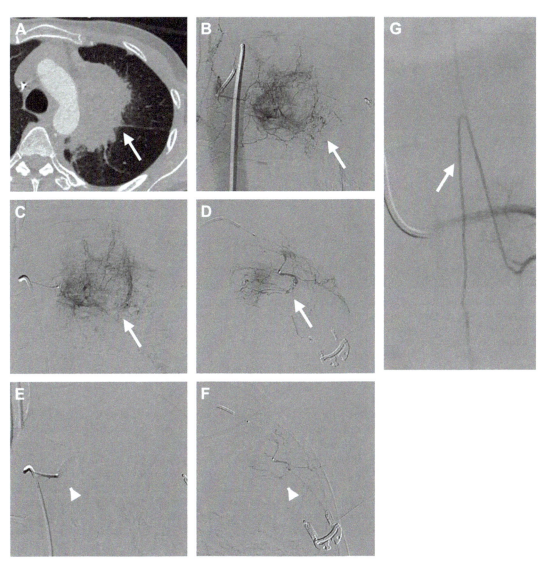

Fig. 5. Bronchial artery embolization for massive hemoptysis. (*A*) Chest CT reveals a central left lung mass with no active extravasation (*arrow*). (*B–D*) Arteriography demonstrates tumor supply via left bronchial (*arrow, B, C*) and lateral thoracic arterial branches (*arrow, D*). (*E, F*) After particle embolization, there is pruning of tumor hypervascularity (*arrowheads*). (*G*) The anterior spinal artery (*arrow*) arises from an incidentally catheterized T8 intercostal artery.

negative bronchial arteriography for massive hemoptysis may reasonably undergo pulmonary arteriography as a next step.[63,64] While thoracotomy and resection of the injured region provides definitive management, endovascular intervention is an effective, minimally invasive alternative.[63]

Contraindications are limited to those discussed for pulmonary DSA.[65] PA embolization is a low-bleeding-risk procedure, with a platelet threshold of greater than 20,000 and INR less than 2.0 to 3.0.[1] As patients often present with massive hemoptysis, intervention under general anesthesia is advisable; dual-lumen intubation can be considered to isolate the unaffected lung.

After jugular or femoral venous access and PA catheterization, diagnostic main pulmonary arteriography is performed in multiple projections. The injured vessel is selected using base catheters and microcatheters, if needed. The goal in treatment is permanent pseudoaneurysm or injury occlusion or exclusion; device selection depends on the size and location of the injury and operator comfort, with options including coils, plugs, liquid embolics such as glue or Onyx (Medtronic PLC, Minneapolis, MN), or stent-grafts. If the area of injury can be embolized, care should be taken to embolize across the area of injury to prevent retrograde filling from aberrant PA collaterals (**Fig. 6**C

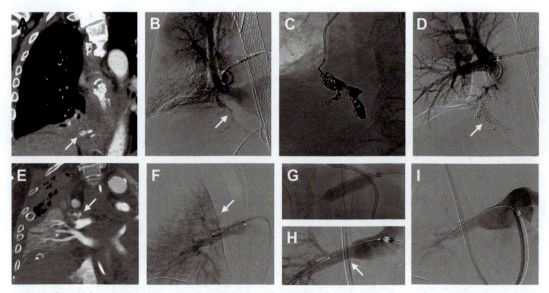

Fig. 6. Endovascular interventions in pulmonary artery hemorrhage. (*A, B*) Contrast-enhanced chest CT and pulmonary angiography reveal subsegmental pulmonary artery pseudoaneurysm in a patient with bloody drain output after thoracotomy and esophageal stenting (*arrows*). (*C, D*) After coil embolization, there is no residual pseudoaneurysm filling (*arrows*). (*E, F*) Contrast-enhanced chest CT and pulmonary angiography reveal PA anastomotic dehiscence in a lung transplant recipient with massive hemoptysis (*arrows*). (*G–I*) After balloon-expandable stent-graft deployment, there is no residual extravasation and preserved filling of distal pulmonary artery branches (*arrows*).

and D).[64] If the injured area is proximal, such as in a main PA, covered stent deployment is reasonable to avoid vessel sacrifice (**Fig. 6**G-I).[62,66] Post-treatment angiography is performed to confirm occlusion or exclusion of the injury.

Assessment of safety and efficacy of endovascular management of pulmonary arterial hemorrhage is limited by the lack of large case series, though a review of 41 patients with post-Swan-Ganz catheter PA pseudoaneurysms demonstrated coil embolization technical success in 89% of the cases.[67] Complications can include embolic migration, nontarget embolization, and parent or branch vessel occlusion leading to pulmonary infarct.[67]

FOREIGN BODY RETRIEVAL

Patients with indwelling vascular implants or undergoing endovascular procedures are at risk for foreign body embolization. While removal historically required operative intervention, minimally invasive endovascular retrieval of embolized foreign bodies is now standard of care.[68] Unintended embolization or migration of a foreign body is generally an indication for attempted retrieval, as complications of embolization include infection, vessel occlusion, ischemia, or vessel/myocardial injury.[68] Small, distally-embolized fragments that are clinically inconsequential may not require retrieval. Endovascular removal of foreign bodies in which the risks of removal outweigh the benefits should also be deferred, and multidisciplinary management should be considered in these cases. Foreign body retrieval may be either a low-bleeding-risk or high-bleeding-risk procedure depending on the vasculature and sheath sizes involved, and coagulation parameters should be corrected accordingly.[1]

For devices that have embolized to the superior or inferior vena cavae, right heart, or pulmonary arteries, IJ or CFV access is obtained. After placement of a sheath large enough to accommodate the foreign body, endovascular snares or forceps may be advanced to the embolized body under fluoroscopic guidance, and an available loose end may be snared and retrieved (**Fig. 7**A and B). If the embolized body is linear but has no easily snared end, more advanced techniques are available, including using shaped catheters, wires, and/or balloons to entangle, pull, or push the embolized body into a position more amenable for retrieval (**Fig. 7**C).[68] Once secured, the foreign body is removed through the sheath. Thorough completion images should be obtained to ensure the foreign body is entirely removed (**Fig. 7**D).

While data from large studies is limited, reported foreign body retrieval technical success ranges from 90% to 100%, and reported overall survival of attempted endovascular foreign body retrieval is 100%.[68,69] Complications include foreign body

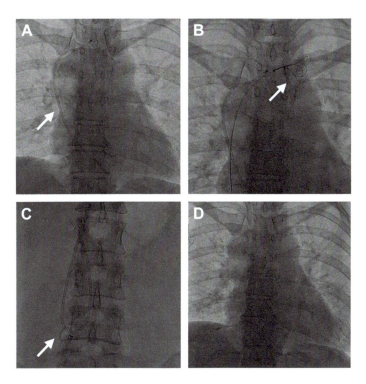

Fig. 7. Endovascular foreign body retrieval techniques. (*A*) A port catheter fragment embolized to the left brachiocephalic vein, superior vena cava, and right heart (*arrow*). (*B*) A trilobed snare (*arrow*) advanced from a right common femoral vein sheath was unable to snare the free end of the catheter. (*C*) A pigtail catheter was used to entangle and retract the catheter fragment into the inferior vena cava (*arrow*); a free end of the catheter was subsequently snared and the catheter removed. (*D*) Final imaging shows complete removal of the catheter fragment.

fragmentation and further embolization, arrhythmias, vessel injury or occlusion, or myocardial injury. If endovascular retrieval fails and foreign body removal remains indicated, operative removal may be considered, and multidisciplinary discussions should be considered in this setting.

SUMMARY

Endovascular intervention is a safe and effective treatment modality in the management of a wide range of pulmonary vascular pathologies, including acute or chronic thromboembolic disease, pulmonary arteriovenous malformations, pulmonary artery or bronchial artery hemorrhage, and foreign body retrieval. Familiarity with the indications, contraindications, techniques, and outcomes of endovascular management is critical for contemporary interventional radiologists.

CLINICS CARE POINTS

- Minimally invasive endovascular techniques have largely replaced operative management of pulmonary vascular diseases and are often appropriate for management of acute and chronic PE; infectious, inflammatory, or post-traumatic pulmonary vascular injuries; pAVMs; and embolized foreign bodies.

- Diagnostic pulmonary arteriography is a mainstay of pulmonary arterial interventions, and multiplanar arteriography and pressure measurements facilitate diagnosis and intervention.

- Pulmonary artery interventions, including mechanical or pharmacomechanical thrombectomy or catheter-based thrombolysis, may be indicated in acute massive or submassive PE. Treatment decisions should be made in a multidisciplinary setting.

- Balloon pulmonary angioplasty may be indicated in CTEPH. Treatment decisions should be made in a multidisciplinary, high-volume setting, and interventions performed at experienced centers.

- Embolization should be performed in all pAVMs visible by imaging, with occlusion of the pAVM nidus and all feeding vessels.

- Endovascular techniques for management of hemoptysis vary according to underlying etiology and culprit vessels.

DISCLOSURES

The authors have no relevant disclosures.

REFERENCES

1. Patel IJ, Rahim S, Davidson JC, et al. Society of Interventional Radiology Consensus Guidelines for the

1. Periprocedural Management of Thrombotic and Bleeding Risk in Patients Undergoing Percutaneous Image-Guided Interventions-Part II: Recommendations: Endorsed by the Canadian Association for Interventional Radiology and the Cardiovascular and Interventional Radiological Society of Europe. J Vasc Interv Radiol 2019;30(8):1168–1184 e1.
2. Valji K. The practice of interventional radiology: with online cases and videos. 2nd edition. Philadelphia, PA: Elsevier; 2012.
3. Nilsson T, Carlsson A, Mare K. Pulmonary angiography: a safe procedure with modern contrast media and technique. Eur Radiol 1998;8(1):86–9.
4. Broaddus VC, Ernst JD, King TE Jr, et al. Murray & Nadel's textbook of respiratory medicine. 7th edition. Philadelphia, PA: Elsevier; 2022. 2 volumes (xli, 1993, I-81 pages).
5. Xue X, Sista AK. Catheter-directed thrombolysis for pulmonary embolism: the state of practice. Tech Vasc Interv Radiol 2018;21(2):78–84.
6. Jaff MR, McMurtry MS, Archer SL, et al. Management of massive and submassive pulmonary embolism, iliofemoral deep vein thrombosis, and chronic thromboembolic pulmonary hypertension: a scientific statement from the American Heart Association. Circulation 2011;123(16):1788–830.
7. Stevens SM, Woller SC, Kreuziger LB, et al. Antithrombotic therapy for VTE disease: second update of the CHEST guideline and expert panel report. Chest 2021;160(6):e545–608.
8. Gotzinger F, Lauder L, Sharp ASP, et al. Interventional therapies for pulmonary embolism. Nat Rev Cardiol 2023;20(10):670–84.
9. Harvey JJ, Huang S, Uberoi R. Catheter-directed therapies for the treatment of high risk (massive) and intermediate risk (submassive) acute pulmonary embolism. Cochrane Database Syst Rev 2022;8(8):CD013083.
10. Sadeghipour P, Jenab Y, Moosavi J, et al. Catheter-directed thrombolysis vs anticoagulation in patients with acute intermediate-high-risk pulmonary embolism: the CANARY randomized clinical trial. JAMA Cardiol 2022;7(12):1189–97.
11. Avgerinos ED, Jaber W, Lacomis J, et al. Randomized trial comparing standard versus ultrasound-assisted thrombolysis for submassive pulmonary embolism: the SUNSET sPE trial. JACC Cardiovasc Interv 2021;14(12):1364–73.
12. Kucher N, Boekstegers P, Muller OJ, et al. Randomized, controlled trial of ultrasound-assisted catheter-directed thrombolysis for acute intermediate-risk pulmonary embolism. Circulation 2014;129(4):479–86.
13. Tapson VF, Sterling K, Jones N, et al. A randomized trial of the optimum duration of acoustic pulse thrombolysis procedure in acute intermediate-risk pulmonary embolism: the OPTALYSE PE trial. JACC Cardiovasc Interv 2018;11(14):1401–10.
14. Piazza G, Hohlfelder B, Jaff MR, et al. A prospective, single-arm, multicenter trial of ultrasound-facilitated, catheter-directed, low-dose fibrinolysis for acute massive and submassive pulmonary embolism: the SEATTLE II study. JACC Cardiovasc Interv 2015;8(10):1382–92.
15. Tu T, Toma C, Tapson VF, et al. A prospective, single-arm, multicenter trial of catheter-directed mechanical thrombectomy for intermediate-risk acute pulmonary embolism: the FLARE study. JACC Cardiovasc Interv 2019;12(9):859–69.
16. Toma C, Bunte MC, Cho KH, et al. Percutaneous mechanical thrombectomy in a real-world pulmonary embolism population: Interim results of the FLASH registry. Catheter Cardiovasc Interv 2022;99(4):1345–55.
17. Toma C, Jaber WA, Weinberg MD, et al. Acute outcomes for the full US cohort of the FLASH mechanical thrombectomy registry in pulmonary embolism. EuroIntervention 2023;18(14):1201–12.
18. Sista AK, Horowitz JM, Tapson VF, et al. Indigo aspiration system for treatment of pulmonary embolism: results of the EXTRACT-PE trial. JACC Cardiovasc Interv 2021;14(3):319–29.
19. Konstantinides SV, Meyer G, Becattini C, et al. 2019 ESC Guidelines for the diagnosis and management of acute pulmonary embolism developed in collaboration with the European Respiratory Society (ERS). Eur Heart J 2020;41(4):543–603.
20. Braaten JV, Goss RA, Francis CW. Ultrasound reversibly disaggregates fibrin fibers. Thromb Haemost 1997;78(3):1063–8.
21. Owens CA. Ultrasound-enhanced thrombolysis: EKOS EndoWave infusion catheter system. Semin Intervent Radiol 2008;25(1):37–41.
22. Bashir R, Foster M, Iskander A, et al. Pharmacomechanical catheter-directed thrombolysis with the bashir endovascular catheter for acute pulmonary embolism: the RESCUE study. JACC Cardiovasc Interv 2022;15(23):2427–36.
23. Phan K, Jo HE, Xu J, et al. Medical therapy versus balloon angioplasty for CTEPH: a systematic review and meta-analysis. Heart Lung Circ 2018;27(1):89–98.
24. Higuchi S, Horinouchi H, Aoki T, et al. Balloon pulmonary angioplasty in the management of chronic thromboembolic pulmonary hypertension. Radiographics 2022;42(6):1881–96.
25. Humbert M, Kovacs G, Hoeper MM, et al. 2022 ESC/ERS Guidelines for the diagnosis and treatment of pulmonary hypertension. Eur Respir J 2023;61(1):2200879.
26. Kawakami T, Matsubara H, Shinke T, et al. Balloon pulmonary angioplasty versus riociguat in inoperable chronic thromboembolic pulmonary hypertension (MR BPA): an open-label, randomised controlled trial. Lancet Respir Med 2022;10(10):949–60.

27. Sugimura K, Fukumoto Y, Satoh K, et al. Percutaneous transluminal pulmonary angioplasty markedly improves pulmonary hemodynamics and long-term prognosis in patients with chronic thromboembolic pulmonary hypertension. Circ J 2012;76(2):485–8.
28. Darocha S, Pietura R, Pietrasik A, et al. Improvement in quality of life and hemodynamics in chronic thromboembolic pulmonary hypertension treated with balloon pulmonary angioplasty. Circ J 2017;81(4):552–7.
29. Zoppellaro G, Badawy MR, Squizzato A, et al. Balloon pulmonary angioplasty in patients with chronic thromboembolic pulmonary hypertension - a systematic review and meta-analysis. Circ J 2019;83(8):1660–7.
30. Ogo T. Balloon pulmonary angioplasty for inoperable chronic thromboembolic pulmonary hypertension. Curr Opin Pulm Med 2015;21(5):425–31.
31. Lang I, Meyer BC, Ogo T, et al. Balloon pulmonary angioplasty in chronic thromboembolic pulmonary hypertension. Eur Respir Rev 2017;26(143):160119.
32. Mahmud E, Behnamfar O, Ang L, et al. Balloon pulmonary angioplasty for chronic thromboembolic pulmonary hypertension. Interv Cardiol Clin 2018;7(1):103–17.
34. Rihal CS, Raphael C. Elsevier handbook of structural heart interventionsxii. Philadelphia, PA: Elsevier; 2021. p. 388. illustrations (chiefly colour).
34. Kataoka M, Inami T, Hayashida K, et al. Percutaneous transluminal pulmonary angioplasty for the treatment of chronic thromboembolic pulmonary hypertension. Circ Cardiovasc Interv 2012;5(6):756–62.
35. Inami T, Kataoka M, Shimura N, et al. Pulmonary edema predictive scoring index (PEPSI), a new index to predict risk of reperfusion pulmonary edema and improvement of hemodynamics in percutaneous transluminal pulmonary angioplasty. JACC Cardiovasc Interv 2013;6(7):725–36.
36. Delcroix M, Torbicki A, Gopalan D, et al. ERS statement on chronic thromboembolic pulmonary hypertension. Eur Respir J 2021;57(6):2002828.
37. Feinstein JA, Goldhaber SZ, Lock JE, et al. Balloon pulmonary angioplasty for treatment of chronic thromboembolic pulmonary hypertension. Circulation 2001;103(1):10–3.
38. Brenot P, Jais X, Taniguchi Y, et al. French experience of balloon pulmonary angioplasty for chronic thromboembolic pulmonary hypertension. Eur Respir J 2019;53(5):1802095.
39. Majumdar S, McWilliams JP. Approach to pulmonary arteriovenous malformations: a comprehensive update. J Clin Med 2020;9(6):1927.
40. Hsu CC, Kwan GN, Evans-Barns H, et al. Embolisation for pulmonary arteriovenous malformation. Cochrane Database Syst Rev 2018;1(1):CD008017.
41. Faughnan ME, Palda VA, Garcia-Tsao G, et al. International guidelines for the diagnosis and management of hereditary haemorrhagic telangiectasia. J Med Genet 2011;48(2):73–87.
42. Shovlin CL, Jackson JE, Bamford KB, et al. Primary determinants of ischaemic stroke/brain abscess risks are independent of severity of pulmonary arteriovenous malformations in hereditary haemorrhagic telangiectasia. Thorax 2008;63(3):259–66.
43. Lee SY, Lee J, Kim YH, et al. Efficacy and safety of AMPLATZER vascular plug type IV for embolization of pulmonary arteriovenous malformations. J Vasc Interv Radiol 2019;30(7):1082–8.
44. Shimohira M, Kawai T, Hashizume T, et al. Reperfusion rates of pulmonary arteriovenous malformations after coil embolization: evaluation with time-resolved MR angiography or pulmonary angiography. J Vasc Interv Radiol 2015;26(6):856–864 e1.
45. Stein EJ, Chittams JL, Miller M, et al. Persistence in coil-embolized pulmonary arteriovenous malformations with feeding artery diameters of 3 mm or less: a retrospective single-center observational study. J Vasc Interv Radiol 2017;28(3):442–9.
46. Ratnani R, Sutphin PD, Koshti V, et al. Retrospective comparison of pulmonary arteriovenous malformation embolization with the polytetrafluoroethylene-covered nitinol microvascular plug, AMPLATZER plug, and coils in patients with hereditary hemorrhagic telangiectasia. J Vasc Interv Radiol 2019;30(7):1089–97.
47. Chamarthy MR, Park H, Sutphin P, et al. Pulmonary arteriovenous malformations: endovascular therapy. Cardiovasc Diagn Ther 2018;8(3):338–49.
48. Trerotola SO, Pyeritz RE. Does use of coils in addition to amplatzer vascular plugs prevent recanalization? AJR Am J Roentgenol 2010;195(3):766–71.
49. Hayashi S, Baba Y, Senokuchi T, et al. Efficacy of venous sac embolization for pulmonary arteriovenous malformations: comparison with feeding artery embolization. J Vasc Interv Radiol 2012;23(12): 1566–77. quiz p 1581.
50. Cusumano LR, Duckwiler GR, Roberts DG, et al. Treatment of recurrent pulmonary arteriovenous malformations: comparison of proximal versus distal embolization technique. Cardiovasc Intervent Radiol 2020;43(1):29–36.
51. Kennedy SA, Faughnan ME, Vozoris NT, et al. Reperfusion of pulmonary arteriovenous malformations following embolotherapy: a randomized controlled trial of detachable versus pushable coils. Cardiovasc Intervent Radiol 2020;43(6):904–9.
52. Prasad V, Chan RP, Faughnan ME. Embolotherapy of pulmonary arteriovenous malformations: efficacy of platinum versus stainless steel coils. J Vasc Interv Radiol 2004;15(2 Pt 1):153–60.
53. Fidelman N, Gordon RL, Bloom AI, et al. Reperfusion of pulmonary arteriovenous malformations after successful embolotherapy with vascular plugs. J Vasc Interv Radiol 2008;19(8):1246–50.
54. Milic A, Chan RP, Cohen JH, et al. Reperfusion of pulmonary arteriovenous malformations after embolotherapy. J Vasc Interv Radiol 2005;16(12):1675–83.

55. Kucukay F, Topcuoglu OM, Alpar A, et al. Bronchial artery embolization with large sized (700-900 microm) Tris-acryl microspheres (Embosphere) for massive hemoptysis: long-term results (Clinical Research). Cardiovasc Intervent Radiol 2018;41(2): 225–30.
56. Hwang JH, Kim JH, Park S, et al. Feasibility and outcomes of bronchial artery embolization in patients with non-massive hemoptysis. Respir Res 2021; 22(1):221.
57. Panda A, Bhalla AS, Goyal A. Bronchial artery embolization in hemoptysis: a systematic review. Diagn Interv Radiol 2017;23(4):307–17.
58. Corr PD. Bronchial artery embolization for life-threatening hemoptysis using tris-acryl microspheres: short-term result. Cardiovasc Intervent Radiol 2005;28(4):439–41.
59. Dave BR, Sharma A, Kalva SP, et al. Nine-year single-center experience with transcatheter arterial embolization for hemoptysis: medium-term outcomes. Vasc Endovascular Surg 2011;45(3): 258–68.
60. Chun JY, Morgan R, Belli AM. Radiological management of hemoptysis: a comprehensive review of diagnostic imaging and bronchial arterial embolization. Cardiovasc Intervent Radiol 2010;33(2): 240–50.
61. Chan VL, So LK, Lam JY, et al. Major haemoptysis in Hong Kong: aetiologies, angiographic findings and outcomes of bronchial artery embolisation. Int J Tuberc Lung Dis 2009;13(9):1167–73.
62. Barrot V, Pellerin O, Reverdito G, et al. Ruptured pulmonary artery pseudoaneurysm treated with stent graft: case report and literature review. CVIR Endovasc 2022;5(1):59.
63. Pelage JP, El Hajjam M, Lagrange C, et al. Pulmonary artery interventions: an overview. Radiographics 2005;25(6):1653–67.
64. Santelli ED, Katz DS, Goldschmidt AM, et al. Embolization of multiple Rasmussen aneurysms as a treatment of hemoptysis. Radiology 1994;193(2):396–8.
65. Chou MC, Liang HL, Pan HB, et al. Percutaneous stent-graft repair of a mycotic pulmonary artery pseudoaneurysm. Cardiovasc Intervent Radiol 2006;29(5):890–2.
66. Klobuka AJ, Short RF. Endovascular stent graft placement in the left main pulmonary artery for management of a giant pulmonary artery pseudoaneurysm. J Vasc Interv Radiol 2016;27(11):1706–7.
67. Nellaiyappan M, Omar HR, Justiz R, et al. Pulmonary artery pseudoaneurysm after Swan-Ganz catheterization: a case presentation and review of literature. Eur Heart J Acute Cardiovasc Care 2014;3(3): 281–8.
68. Woodhouse JB, Uberoi R. Techniques for intravascular foreign body retrieval. Cardiovasc Intervent Radiol 2013;36(4):888–97.
69. Leite TFO, Pazinato LV, Bortolini E, et al. Endovascular removal of intravascular foreign bodies: a single-center experience and literature review. Ann Vasc Surg 2022;82:362–76.

The Role of Imaging in Pulmonary Vascular Disease: The Clinician's Perspective

Brandon R. Jakubowski, MD[a], Megan Griffiths, MD[b], Kara N. Goss, MD[a,b,*]

KEYWORDS

- Pulmonary hypertension • Pulmonary vascular diseases • Right ventricle • Pulmonary artery
- Cardiac MR imaging • Computed tomography • Ventilation perfusion scintigraphy

KEY POINTS

- Pulmonary vascular diseases, particularly when accompanied by pulmonary hypertension, are complex disorders that require multimodal imaging for diagnosis and subsequent monitoring.
- Although invasive right heart catheterization is required for definitive diagnosis and essential in pulmonary arterial hypertension, most patients with mild pulmonary hypertension never undergo catheterization. Rather, clinicians rely heavily on noninvasive cardiac and pulmonary vascular imaging studies to classify and risk-stratify patients.
- Mortality in pulmonary hypertension is largely determined by right ventricular function, making echocardiography and cardiac MR imaging critical for serial monitoring.

INTRODUCTION

Pulmonary hypertension (PH) is a complex and highly morbid disease characterized by either a primary pulmonary vasculopathy or, more commonly, secondary to pulmonary vascular remodeling due to cardiac, pulmonary, or other systemic conditions.[1] PH is defined hemodynamically by a mean pulmonary artery (PA) pressure of greater than 20 mm Hg and is estimated to affect approximately 1% of the worldwide population. Patients with PH are grouped together based on clinical presentation, pathophysiology, and hemodynamics, with several recent updates to the hemodynamic classifications and thresholds[1] (**Table 1**). The most common causes are due to left heart disease followed by lung disease, while pulmonary arterial hypertension (PAH; Group 1) and chronic thromboembolic pulmonary hypertension (CTEPH; Group 4) are rare. Given the clinical overlap between these groups, multimodal diagnostic evaluation is required.

Although invasive right heart catheterization is required for definitive diagnosis and essential in PAH, most patients with mild PH never undergo catheterization. Rather, clinicians rely heavily on noninvasive imaging to classify and risk-stratify patients. Echocardiography is the most widely employed imaging modality for screening for PH and provides initial clues to etiology and severity. Integration of additional imaging modalities is necessary in the comprehensive evaluation of PH.[1,2] Cardiac MR imaging (CMR) provides additional diagnostic assessment and risk stratification of right ventricular (RV) failure. Computed tomography (CT) and ventilation/perfusion (V/Q) scintigraphy allow for assessment of the pulmonary and mediastinal structures as well as pulmonary blood flow. Pulmonary angiography can supplement these modalities and is primarily used in the workup of CTEPH, as well as in the evaluation of pulmonary arteriovenous malformations, pulmonary stenosis, and intrapulmonary shunts. Understanding

---

[a] Department of Medicine, UT Southwestern Medical Center, 5323 Harry Hines Boulevard, Dallas, TX 75390-8558, USA; [b] Department of Pediatrics, UT Southwestern Medical Center, 5323 Harry Hines Boulevard, Dallas, TX 75390-8558, USA
* Corresponding author.
E-mail address: kara.goss@utsouthwestern.edu

Table 1
Overview of pulmonary hypertension classification and characteristic imaging findings

PH Group	Common Clinical Etiologies	Hemodynamic Definition	Characteristic Imaging Findings
Group 1	Idiopathic PAH Hereditable PAH Drug/toxin PAH CTD associated PAH Porto-pulmonary hypertension Congenital heart disease PVOD	mPAP >20 mm Hg PAWP ≤15 mm Hg PVR >2 WU	• CT with centrilobular nodules, peripheral neovascularization, and lobular areas of ground-glass attenuation • Dilated right atrium, right ventricle, pulmonary artery
Group 2	HFpEF HFrEF Valvular heart disease	mPAP >20 mm Hg PAWP >15 mm Hg	• Left atrial and ventricular enlargement/hypertrophy • Pleural effusions, pulmonary edema
Group 3	Lung diseases, that is, COPD, ILD Developmental lung diseases Hypoxia Hypoventilation syndromes	mPAP >20 mm Hg PAWP ≤15 mm Hg	• CXR or CT parenchymal abnormalities consistent with lung disease • Dilated pulmonary artery
Group 4	CTEPH Other pulmonary artery obstructions	mPAP >20 mm Hg PAWP ≤15 mm Hg PVR >2 WU	• Mismatched perfusion defects on VQ • Filling defects, webs, bands on CTA
Group 5	Unclear or multifactorial mechanisms, clinically includes myeloproliferative disorders, metabolic disorders, sarcoidosis, Langerhans cell histiocytosis, neurofibromatosis, fibrosing mediastinitis, ESRD	Varies by etiology	Varies by etiology

Abbreviations: CTEPH, chronic thromboembolic pulmonary hypertension; COPD, chronic obstructive pulmonary disease; CTD, connective tissue disease; ESRD, end-stage renal disease; HFrEF, heart failure with reduced ejection fraction; HFpEF, heart failure with preserved ejection fraction; ILD, interstitial lung disease; mPAP, mean pulmonary artery pressure; PAWP, pulmonary artery wedge pressure; PVOD, pulmonary veno-occlusive disease; PVR, pulmonary vascular resistance.

the advantages and disadvantages these available tools is critical for the diagnosis and follow-up of patients with PH. Insights gained by these imaging studies enhance our understanding of the physiology of pulmonary vascular disease. This review focuses on the clinical use of key imaging modalities in pulmonary vascular diseases, particularly PH, for proper classification, risk assessment, and treatment.

ECHOCARDIOGRAPHY

Echocardiography is the primary imaging modality for both the initial diagnosis and serial follow-up of PH. It is a widely available, reliable, and cost-effective tool to evaluate cardiac structure and function. Guidelines recommend echocardiography to screen for PH, with the probability of PH based on tricuspid regurgitant velocity (TRV) and other echocardiographic findings.[1] RV systolic pressure measured using Doppler of the TRV is used to estimate PA systolic pressure. A TRV greater than 3.4 m/s suggests a high probability of PH, while a TRV less than 2.8 m/s suggests a low probability.[1] This method relies on an adequate acoustic window, appropriate Doppler beam alignment, as well as sufficient tricuspid regurgitation for an adequate Doppler envelope to estimate TRV and thus is not achievable in all patients. The initial screening echocardiogram also includes a comprehensive evaluation of cardiac structures (valves, atrial and ventricular septum, etc.) and function, which can provide clues as to the origin of PH. Evaluation of the left ventricle (LV) for left heart disease is essential for diagnosing Group 2 PH.[3] Based on this initial screening, further imaging and diagnostic cardiac catheterization are pursued.

Several features beyond TRV suggest PH, many of which are also visible on other imaging modalities more commonly interpreted by radiologists. Measurement of the RV volume in systole and diastole in the 4 chamber view can be used to calculate a fractional area change (FAC) as a quantitative measure of RV systolic function, where a FAC less than 35% indicates RV systolic dysfunction.[4] Right atrial (RA) area should be calculated from the 4 chamber view, as an RA area greater than 26 cm^2 predicts a poor outcome.[4] The basal dimensions of the RV and LV in the 4 chamber or parasternal short axis views should be compared, with an elevated RV:LV ratio strongly associated with worse outcomes.[5] In adults, an RV:LV dimension greater than 1 is considered abnormal, while in pediatrics, an increasing RV:LV ratio predicts progressively worse outcomes.[6,7] Flattening of the interventricular septum, often termed a "D-shaped septum," is a strong indicator of RV pressure overload and suggests PH. Any of these findings require additional diagnostic evaluation.

For patients with PH, risk stratification models such as the (Registry to Evaluate Early and Long-Term PAH Disease Management [REVEAL]) 2.0 score and the European Respiratory Society risk criteria include multiple echocardiographic parameters of RV size and function.[1,8] RA area, tricuspid annular plane systolic excursion, and presence of a pericardial effusion continue to show the best prognostic value and are used for risk assessment. Presence and size of a pericardial effusion should always be documented as this remains one of the best indicators of RV failure and may require aggressive acute management.[9] Serial echocardiograms are used to guide therapy with the goal being to target low risk status for the best long-term prognosis.[10,11]

CARDIAC MR IMAGING

Cardiac MR imaging (CMR) is considered the reference-standard for imaging the RV. While CMR is not used routinely for the initial diagnosis of PH in many centers, its superior resolution and characterization of cardiac structure and function allow for precise and repeatable evaluations of RV function, volumes, and mass. Clinically, CMR is frequently used for evaluation of cardiac diseases associated with PH (eg, congenital heart disease and infiltrative cardiomyopathies) and serially for risk stratification and response to medical therapy. Steady-state free-precession sequences provide accurate analysis of biventricular structure and function, classically showing RV dilation and hypertrophy. Septal bowing and left atrial (LA) or LV compression suggest RV pressure overload states commonly seen in PAH. Late gadolinium enhancement (LGE) frequently identifies increased collagen deposition at the RV insertion points, with greater mass of LGE associated with worse hemodynamic profiles in PAH.[12] LA or LV dilation, reduced LV ejection fraction, and impaired LV diastolic function suggest Group 2 PH. Two dimensional phase-contrast imaging is used to assess PA hemodynamics, including mean PA velocity, pulse wave velocity, and relative area change, all markers of PA stiffness. Proximal PA stiffness, assessed by PA relative area change from systole to diastole, also predicts increased mortality risk in PAH.[13] Additional novel metrics capture PA–RV mechanical coupling, a measure of RV contractile function relative to afterload, and are also associated with increased mortality risk. The most utilized index in CMR is a volumetric method defined as RV stroke volume/RV end-systolic volume, though measures of LV eccentricity and RV strain are increasingly utilized to assess ventricular–vascular coupling.[14–16]

RV failure is a key determinant of prognosis and mortality in PH, and CMR is included many risk assessment models. CMR is also used to define treatment-associated functional recovery in patients with PAH and is more sensitive than classically followed PAH outcome parameters such as 6 min walk distance and (N-terminal pro b-type natriuretic peptide [NT-proBNP]).[17,18] A meta-analysis of 22 studies by Alabed and colleagues demonstrated that every 1% decrease in RV ejection fraction was associated with a 4.9% increase in risk for clinical worsening (defined as hospitalization, disease progression, or mortality) and a 2.1% increased risk of death. Further, a 1 mL/m^2 increase in RV end-systolic volume index or RV end-diastolic volume index increased risk of clinical worsening by 1.3% and 1%, respectively.[19] With respect to treatment response, a 5% absolute increase in RV ejection fraction and a 17 mL decrease in RV end-diastolic or end-systolic volumes were identified as the minimally important differences associated with improvement in overall patient symptoms, daily functioning, and survival. However, a 5% decrease in RV ejection fraction or 10 mL increase in RV volumes was associated with clinical worsening.[20] A recent study also suggested 1 year follow-up CMR-based risk assessment is at least non-inferior to invasive catheterization-based risk assessment, supporting its growing use.[21]

Other novel applications of CMR in PH include use of PET/MR imaging to assess myocardial metabolism,[22–24] simultaneous measurement of invasive hemodynamics,[25] and application of in-scanner exercise programs.[23] Novel multi-parametric CMR models are now being used to estimate mean PA pressure with reasonable diagnostic accuracy, though these methods have not yet reached clinical practice. Furthermore, the ability to distinguish high versus low pulmonary capillary wedge pressure (and thus PAH from Group 2 PH or mixed PH) will be critical if CMR is to supplant right heart catheterization.[26]

CHEST RADIOGRAPHY

While chest radiography has a limited role in elucidating the etiology of pulmonary vascular disease, it remains an important and cost-effective tool to suggest need for additional evaluation. Frequently abnormal at the time of initial diagnosis, chest radiographs may show an enlarged cardiac silhouette, PA dilation, or pruning of peripheral vessels.[1,2] The identification of Kerley B lines or pleural effusion may prompt consideration of pulmonary venous hypertension due to left heart disease (Group 2 PH), while significant reticulation or emphysema may suggest PH due to lung disease (Group 3 PH). The utility of chest radiography should not be underestimated, particularly in resource-poor settings where more advanced imaging modalities may be less accessible.

COMPUTED TOMOGRAPHY

CT has secured a crucial position in the evaluation of pulmonary vascular disease. It offers a swift assessment of cardiac, mediastinal, vascular, and pulmonary structures, using high-spatial-resolution isovolumetric imaging. Three CT variations are commonly used in contemporary practice: unenhanced CT imaging, CT angiography (CTA), and high-resolution CT imaging (HRCT). In this section, we will also review dual-energy CT (DECT) and single photon emission computed tomography (SPECT) as imaging techniques with evolving utility.

Unenhanced Computed Tomography and High-resolution Computed Tomography

Distinct abnormalities may be indicative of specific disorders and have notably unique imaging findings on unenhanced and HRCT images. These include signs of emphysema, interstitial lung disease, pulmonary Langerhans cell histiocytosis, or pulmonary sarcoidosis, all of which can lead to PH. An anatomic assessment using HRCT can aid in the severity of underlying lung disease, though there is no significant correlation between mean PA pressures and the extent of parenchymal lung disease or fibrosis seen on CT imaging.[27] There are several features and characteristic findings on CT that must be highlighted given their presence in Group 1 PAH, including the development of centrilobular nodules, peripheral neovascularization, and lobular areas of ground-glass attenuation.

Computed Tomography Angiography

CT pulmonary angiography (CTPA) is a specialized application of CT scans in which contrast administration is precisely timed to enhance opacification of the pulmonary arteries. Often completed for evaluation of dyspnea or hemoptysis, features suggestive of PH include the following: PA dilation, tortuosity of the PAs, rapid tapering of the PAs, mosaic attenuation of the lung parenchyma, contiguous reflux of contrast into the inferior vena cava, RV dilation, RV hypertrophy, flattening of the intraventricular septum, and dilation of the bronchial arteries (Fig. 1).[2,28,29]

The PA diameter and the PA to aorta ratio (PA:Ao) have been evaluated as surrogate measures for PH. The initial Framingham study established the upper limit of normal diameter of the PA as measured on CT of 27 mm for female individuals and 29 mm for male individuals.[30] A PA:Ao greater than 1 was 70% sensitive and 92% specific for a mean pulmonary artery pressure greater than 20 mm Hg in one study.[31] However, PA size also reflects disease duration and correlates only moderately with PAP.[32] Thus, while suggestive of PH, additional testing is required to confirm the diagnosis. Combining several CT-derived measures is likely of greater utility as compared to any singular finding alone. A diagnostic model noted by Swift and colleagues[33] combined 3 CT-derived metrics (PA diameter $\geq$30 mm, RV outflow track wall thickness $\geq$6 mm, and septal deviation $\geq$140° [or RV:LV ratio $\geq$1]), which was highly predictive of PH. Spruijt and colleagues[34] noted the addition of ventricular measurements and LV:RV ratio can aid in the predictive performance of CTA in the identification of PAH.

As PH progresses, the pulmonary arterial tree develops increasing levels of vessel tortuosity, which can be quantified through 3 dimensional fractal geometry and has been shown to correlate with mean PA pressure.[35] Additional parameters such as wall thickness and calcification can also indirectly reflect on the stiffness of the PA. Additional benefits of contrast-enhanced CT include the ability to evaluate for other causes of pulmonary vascular disease, including intrapulmonary and extrapulmonary shunts. Acute and chronic thromboembolic disease can also be identified. Characteristic features suggesting chronic disease include thrombus adherent to vessel walls, webs or bands, mosaic attenuation, bronchial artery collateralization, as well as pleural thickening and parenchymal bands. Early differentiation of CTEPH from acute pulmonary embolus (PE) is critical, as while both conditions require anticoagulation, CTEPH is a surgically curable cause of PH

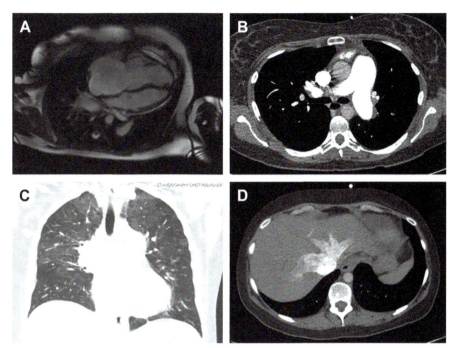

Fig. 1. Characteristic imaging of a patient with Group 1 pulmonary arterial hypertension. Cardiac MR imaging demonstrates a dilated right atrium and dilated, hypertrabeculated right ventricle with septal flattening (A). A small pericardial effusion is present. CTA shows a dilated pulmonary artery (B), peripheral pulmonary arterial pruning, mosaic attenuation of the parenchyma with centrilobular ground glass nodules (C), and reflux of intravenous contrast into the hepatic vasculature suggestive of right ventricular failure (D).

(Fig. 2).[36] Though historically the diagnostic accuracy of CTA for CTEPH had been limited by poor sensitivity, modern scanners have increasing utility and sensitivity compared to prior-generation scanners.

Dual-energy Computed Tomography

DECT simultaneously employs 2 different radiograph energy levels, exploiting the attenuation properties of materials at varying energy levels and enhancing tissue characterization. It provides quantitative analysis of iodine distribution within the pulmonary arteries, providing more functional information regarding perfusion mapping and improved detection of PE. DECT is often used to detect CTEPH, where initial reports demonstrated excellent agreement with lung scintigraphy to identify perfusion defects and differential patterns of acute versus chronic emboli may be seen.[37] In a study of 42 patients, chronic thromboembolic disease was found to have more enhancement based on iodine-related attenuation values on delayed phase imaging than acute embolic segments.[38] DECT perfusion imaging in Group 1 PAH can also demonstrate abnormalities in approximately 50% of patients, though the patterns of perfusion alteration in PAH are typically more homogenous than CTEPH.[39]

Single Photon Emission Computed Tomography

SPECT imaging utilizes gamma-ray-emitting radiotracers and a rotating gamma camera to reconstruct cross-sectional images, assessing pulmonary perfusion. SPECT has higher sensitivity than planar V/Q imaging for detecting thromboemboli, with 97% sensitivity and 91% specificity, and better detects subsegmental defects than CTA by over 80%.[40] In a study on patients with CTEPH undergoing pulmonary thromboendarterectomy, SPECT imaging had a significantly higher sensitivity (64% vs 43%, P<.01) at detecting obstructed lung segments compared to V/Q imaging.[41] Like DECT, SPECT can identify perfusion defects in nonthromboembolic causes of PH, though a majority of these patients demonstrate diffuse, patchy perfusion defects not typical of thromboembolic disease.

VENTILATION/PERFUSION SCINTIGRAPHY

VQ scintigraphy is recommended in the evaluation for all patients with PH.[1] Unfortunately this imaging test has been historically underutilized, leading

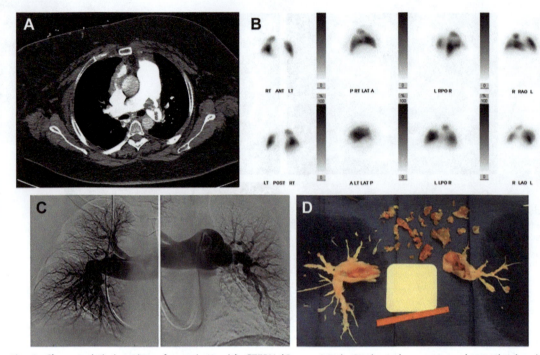

Fig. 2. Characteristic imaging of a patient with CTEPH (Group 4 PH). CT chest demonstrates large clot burden bilaterally, known to be chronic based on serial imaging as well as presence of vascular webs and right ventricular hypertrophy (*A*). Bilateral perfusion defects are present on VQ scan (*B*). Pulmonary angiogram shows diminished perfusion to the right upper and middle lobes with irregularity of distal right pulmonary artery suggesting chronic clot; perfusion on the left lung was severely diminished, with clot extending from the left main pulmonary artery to the lobar artery (*C*). Pulmonary endarterectomy specimen demonstrated extensive bilateral clot from bilateral main pulmonary arteries distally, with large right atrial clot resected in several pieces (*D*).

to the underdiagnosis of CTEPH. Mismatched wedge-shaped segmental defects (ie, lung segments with reduced or absent perfusion but with normal ventilation) are diagnostic for pulmonary embolic disease.[42] A normal V/Q scan effectively excludes CTEPH with a sensitivity of 90% to 100% and a specificity of 94% to 100%.[43,44] In initial studies of confirmed CTEPH, V/Q scan was superior to CTPA with a sensitivity of 97.4% versus 51%.[43] However, more recent studies demonstrated that both V/Q scan and CTPA are accurate methods for the detection of CTEPH with high diagnostic integrity.[44] Though the majority of patients with CTEPH will have frankly abnormal VQ scans consisting of multiple medium-to-large perfusion defects, the size of perfusion defect does not correlate with hemodynamic abnormalities, and physicians should be aware of causes of false-positive results.[45,46]

PULMONARY ANGIOGRAPHY

Current guidelines recommend right-heart catheterization with pulmonary angiography/digital subtraction angiography for patients suspected of having CTEPH with abnormal VQ imaging, given its treatable nature.[1] Angiography is the reference standard for imaging CTEPH, especially when assessing more distal vasculature, as it more readily characterizes vessel morphology. Abnormalities include irregular vessel wall contour, band-like vessel narrowing, weblike structures, vessel pruning, and pouch defects with complete obstruction or absence of large vessels.[47,48] Angiography is crucial for identifying surgically accessible chronic clots or surgically inaccessible distal vessel disease potentially treatable by balloon pulmonary angioplasty.[49]

SPECIAL POPULATIONS
Pulmonary Veno-occlusive Disease/Pulmonary Capillary Hemangiomatosis

Pulmonary veno-occlusive disease/pulmonary capillary hemangiomatosis (PVOD/PCH) deserves special mention. The classic triad of PVOD/PCH CT findings include centrilobular ground-glass nodules, smooth interlobular septal lines, and mediastinal and hilar lymphadenopathy in the absence of pleural effusions (**Fig. 3**).[50,51] A unique clinical feature of PVOD/PCH is the tendency of patients to develop pulmonary edema upon

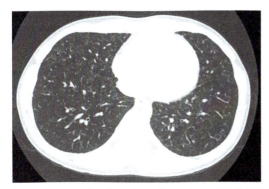

Fig. 3. Characteristic imaging of a patient with PVOD, including the classic triad of centrilobular ground-glass opacities, smooth interlobular septal lines, and mediastinal and hilar lymphadenopathy in the absence of pleural effusions. These patients frequently develop pulmonary edema with pulmonary vasodilator therapy, and thus lung transplant referral should be considered.

initiation of pulmonary vasodilator therapy. Given limited treatment options and high mortality, these findings on imaging should prompt the clinical team to consider early referral for lung transplant evaluation. Because the hemodynamic profile is identical to other forms of Group 1 PAH, the radiologist can play a key role in making the diagnosis when CT findings are characteristic of PVOD/PCH.

Pediatric Populations

Noninvasive imaging also plays a crucial role in diagnosis and management of PH in children. The most common causes of pediatric PH are congenital heart disease and lung disease of prematurity.[52] A comprehensive echocardiogram to evaluate cardiac structure and function is the primary imaging modality in children, as anesthesia is not required. CTA is used to evaluate for airway anomalies, parenchymal lung disease, pulmonary vein stenosis, and other congenital anomalies.[53] Additional imaging modalities may be required to assess for congenital anomalies, such as abdominal ultrasound to screen for arteriovenous malformations, the Abernethy malformation, or hepatic hemangiomas. CMR has an emerging pediatric role to assess cardiac function and pulmonary hemodynamics.[54] CMR fluoroscopy has even been utilized for invasive heart catheterization, avoiding ionizing radiation.[55] Application of free-breathing techniques is reducing the need for sedation during CMR even for the youngest patients, further reducing procedural risk and increasing utilization for serial assessment in pediatric PH.

SUMMARY

In summary, pulmonary vascular diseases, particularly when accompanied by PH, are complex disorders that require multimodal imaging for accurate diagnosis and subsequent monitoring. Clinicians must adeptly apply these modalities for proper management.

CLINICS CARE POINTS

- All patients suspected of having pulmonary hypertension should undergo screening echocardiography.
- Pulmonary hypertension cannot be diagnosed by chest CT imaging. While a dilated pulmonary artery is suggestive of pulmonary hypertension, an echocardiogram or heart catheterization is required.
- Ventilation-perfusion scan remains the preferred imaging modality to diagnose chronic thromboembolic pulmonary hypertension.

DISCLOSURE

K.N. Goss is supported by research funding provided by Southwestern Health Resources Academic Affiliation Committee, and by the National Heart, Lung, And Blood Institute of the National Institutes of Health under Award Number R01HL164853. The content is solely the responsibility of the authors and does not necessarily represent the official views of the National Institutes of Health. The authors have no relevant conflicts of interest.

REFERENCES

1. Humbert M, Kovacs G, Hoeper MM, et al. 2022 ESC/ERS Guidelines for the diagnosis and treatment of pulmonary hypertension: Developed by the task force for the diagnosis and treatment of pulmonary hypertension of the European Society of Cardiology (ESC) and the European Respiratory Society (ERS). Endorsed by the International Society for Heart and Lung Transplantation (ISHLT) and the European Reference Network on rare respiratory diseases (ERN-LUNG). Eur Heart J 2022;43(38):3618–731.
2. Remy-Jardin M, Ryerson CJ, Schiebler ML, et al. Imaging of pulmonary hypertension in adults: a position paper from the Fleischner Society. Eur Respir J 2021;57(1):2004455.
3. Perez VA, Haddad F, Zamanian RT. Diagnosis and management of pulmonary hypertension associated

with left ventricular diastolic dysfunction. Pulm Circ 2012;2(2):163–9.
4. Rudski LG, Lai WW, Afilalo J, et al. Guidelines for the echocardiographic assessment of the right heart in adults: a report from the American Society of Echocardiography endorsed by the European Association of Echocardiography, a registered branch of the European Society of Cardiology, and the Canadian Society of Echocardiography. J Am Soc Echocardiogr 2010;23(7):685–713. ; quiz 786-8.
5. Lang RM, Badano LP, Mor-Avi V, et al. Recommendations for cardiac chamber quantification by echocardiography in adults: an update from the American Society of Echocardiography and the European Association of Cardiovascular Imaging. J Am Soc Echocardiogr 2015;28(1):1–39.e14.
6. Augustine DX, Coates-Bradshaw LD, Willis J, et al. Echocardiographic assessment of pulmonary hypertension: a guideline protocol from the British Society of Echocardiography. Echo Res Pract 2018;5(3):G11–24.
7. Jone PN, Hinzman J, Wagner BD, et al. Right ventricular to left ventricular diameter ratio at end-systole in evaluating outcomes in children with pulmonary hypertension. J Am Soc Echocardiogr 2014;27(2):172–8.
8. Benza RL, Gomberg-Maitland M, Miller DP, et al. The REVEAL Registry risk score calculator in patients newly diagnosed with pulmonary arterial hypertension. Chest 2012;141(2):354–62.
9. Raymond RJ, Hinderliter AL, Willis PW, et al. Echocardiographic predictors of adverse outcomes in primary pulmonary hypertension. J Am Coll Cardiol 2002;39(7):1214–9.
10. Yogeswaran A, Gall H, Fünderich M, et al. Comparison of contemporary risk scores in all groups of pulmonary hypertension: a pulmonary vascular research institute godeep meta-registry analysis, Chest, 2024, S0012-3692(24)00309-X. doi:10.1016/j.chest.2024.03.018.
11. Galiè N, Channick RN, Frantz RP, et al. Risk stratification and medical therapy of pulmonary arterial hypertension. Eur Respir J 2019;53(1):1801889.
12. Kazimierczyk R, Małek ŁA, Szumowski P, et al. Prognostic value of late gadolinium enhancement mass index in patients with pulmonary arterial hypertension. Adv Med Sci 2021;66(1):28–34.
13. Swift AJ, Capener D, Johns C, et al. Magnetic resonance imaging in the prognostic evaluation of patients with pulmonary arterial hypertension. Am J Respir Crit Care Med 2017;196(2):228–39.
14. Vanderpool RR, Pinsky MR, Naeije R, et al. RV-pulmonary arterial coupling predicts outcome in patients referred for pulmonary hypertension. Heart 2015;101(1):37–43.
15. Tello K, Dalmer A, Vanderpool R, et al. Cardiac magnetic resonance imaging-based right ventricular strain analysis for assessment of coupling and diastolic function in pulmonary hypertension. JACC (J Am Coll Cardiol): Cardiovascular Imaging 2019;12(11_Part_1):2155–64.
16. Swift AJ, Wild JM, Nagle SK, et al. Quantitative magnetic resonance imaging of pulmonary hypertension: a practical approach to the current state of the art. J Thorac Imag 2014;29(2):68–79.
17. Rischard FP, Bernardo RJ, Vanderpool RR, et al. Classification and predictors of right ventricular functional recovery in pulmonary arterial hypertension. Circulation Heart failure 2023;16(10):e010555.
18. Swift AJ, Wilson F, Cogliano M, et al. Repeatability and sensitivity to change of non-invasive end points in PAH: the RESPIRE study. Thorax 2021;76(10):1032–5.
19. Alabed S, Shahin Y, Garg P, et al. Cardiac-MRI predicts clinical worsening and mortality in pulmonary arterial hypertension: a systematic review and meta-analysis. JACC Cardiovascular imaging 2021;14(5):931–42.
20. Alabed S, Garg P, Alandejani F, et al. Establishing minimally important differences for cardiac MRI end-points in pulmonary arterial hypertension. Eur Respir J 2023;62(2):2202225.
21. van der Bruggen CE, Handoko ML, Bogaard HJ, et al. The value of hemodynamic measurements or cardiac mri in the follow-up of patients with idiopathic pulmonary arterial hypertension. Chest 2021;159(4):1575–85.
22. Farha S, Saygin D, Park MM, et al. Pulmonary arterial hypertension treatment with carvedilol for heart failure: a randomized controlled trial. JCI insight 2017;2(16):e95240.
23. Barton GP, Corrado PA, Francois CJ, et al. Development of a PET/MRI exercise stress test for determining cardiac glucose dependence in pulmonary arterial hypertension. Pulm Circ 2022;12(1):e12025.
24. Bokhari S, Raina A, Rosenweig EB, et al. PET imaging may provide a novel biomarker and understanding of right ventricular dysfunction in patients with idiopathic pulmonary arterial hypertension. Circ Cardiovasc Imaging 2011;4(6):641–7.
25. Rogers T, Ratnayaka K, Khan JM, et al. CMR fluoroscopy right heart catheterization for cardiac output and pulmonary vascular resistance: results in 102 patients. J Cardiovasc Magn Reson 2016;19(1):54.
26. Johns CS, Kiely DG, Rajaram S, et al. Diagnosis of pulmonary hypertension with cardiac mri: derivation and validation of regression models. Radiology 2019;290(1):61–8.
27. Zisman DA, Karlamangla AS, Ross DJ, et al. High-resolution chest CT findings do not predict the presence of pulmonary hypertension in advanced idiopathic pulmonary fibrosis. Chest 2007;132(3):773–9.
28. Ascha M, Renapurkar RD, Tonelli AR. A review of imaging modalities in pulmonary hypertension. Ann Thorac Med 2017;12(2):61–73.
29. Freed BH, Collins JD, François CJ, et al. MR and CT imaging for the evaluation of pulmonary hypertension. JACC Cardiovascular imaging 2016;9(6):715–32.

30. Truong QA, Massaro JM, Rogers IS, et al. Reference values for normal pulmonary artery dimensions by noncontrast cardiac computed tomography: the Framingham Heart Study. Circ Cardiovasc Imaging 2012;5(1):147–54.
31. Ng CS, Wells AU, Padley SP. A CT sign of chronic pulmonary arterial hypertension: the ratio of main pulmonary artery to aortic diameter. J Thorac Imag 1999;14(4):270–8.
32. Boerrigter B, Mauritz GJ, Marcus JT, et al. Progressive dilatation of the main pulmonary artery is a characteristic of pulmonary arterial hypertension and is not related to changes in pressure. Chest 2010;138(6):1395–401.
33. Swift AJ, Dwivedi K, Johns C, et al. Diagnostic accuracy of CT pulmonary angiography in suspected pulmonary hypertension. Eur Radiol 2020;30(9):4918–29.
34. Spruijt OA, Bogaard HJ, Heijmans MW, et al. Predicting pulmonary hypertension with standard computed tomography pulmonary angiography. Int J Cardiovasc Imaging 2015;31(4):871–9.
35. Helmberger M, Pienn M, Urschler M, et al. Quantification of tortuosity and fractal dimension of the lung vessels in pulmonary hypertension patients. PLoS One 2014;9(1):e87515.
36. Ruggiero A, Screaton NJ. Imaging of acute and chronic thromboembolic disease: state of the art. Clin Radiol 2017;72(5):375–88.
37. Nakazawa T, Watanabe Y, Hori Y, et al. Lung perfused blood volume images with dual-energy computed tomography for chronic thromboembolic pulmonary hypertension: correlation to scintigraphy with single-photon emission computed tomography. J Comput Assist Tomogr 2011;35(5):590–5.
38. Hong YJ, Kim JY, Choe KO, et al. Different perfusion pattern between acute and chronic pulmonary thromboembolism: evaluation with two-phase dual-energy perfusion CT. AJR Am J Roentgenol 2013;200(4):812–7.
39. Giordano J, Khung S, Duhamel A, et al. Lung perfusion characteristics in pulmonary arterial hypertension (PAH) and peripheral forms of chronic thromboembolic pulmonary hypertension (pCTEPH): Dual-energy CT experience in 31 patients. Eur Radiol 2017;27(4):1631–9.
40. Reinartz P, Wildberger JE, Schaefer W, et al. Tomographic imaging in the diagnosis of pulmonary embolism: a comparison between V/Q lung scintigraphy in SPECT technique and multislice spiral CT. J Nucl Med 2004;45(9):1501–8.
41. Soler X, Hoh CK, Test VJ, et al. Single photon emission computed tomography in chronic thromboembolic pulmonary hypertension. Respirology 2011;16(1):131–7.
42. Bajc M, Schümichen C, Grüning T, et al. EANM guideline for ventilation/perfusion single-photon emission computed tomography (SPECT) for diagnosis of pulmonary embolism and beyond. Eur J Nucl Med Mol Imaging 2019;46(12):2429–51.
43. Tunariu N, Gibbs SJ, Win Z, et al. Ventilation-perfusion scintigraphy is more sensitive than multidetector CTPA in detecting chronic thromboembolic pulmonary disease as a treatable cause of pulmonary hypertension. J Nucl Med 2007;48(5):680–4.
44. He J, Fang W, Lv B, et al. Diagnosis of chronic thromboembolic pulmonary hypertension: comparison of ventilation/perfusion scanning and multidetector computed tomography pulmonary angiography with pulmonary angiography. Nucl Med Commun 2012;33(5):459–63.
45. Azarian R, Wartski M, Collignon MA, et al. Lung perfusion scans and hemodynamics in acute and chronic pulmonary embolism. J Nucl Med 1997;38(6):980–3.
46. Gopalan D, Delcroix M, Held M. Diagnosis of chronic thromboembolic pulmonary hypertension. Eur Respir Rev 2017;26(143):851935.
47. Auger WR, Fedullo PF, Moser KM, et al. Chronic major-vessel thromboembolic pulmonary artery obstruction: appearance at angiography. Radiology 1992;182(2):393–8.
48. Kawakami T, Ogawa A, Miyaji K, et al. Novel angiographic classification of each vascular lesion in chronic thromboembolic pulmonary hypertension based on selective angiogram and results of balloon pulmonary angioplasty. Circ Cardiovasc Interv 2016;9(10):e003318.
49. Ang L, McDivit Mizzell A, Daniels LB, et al. Optimal technique for performing invasive pulmonary angiography for chronic thromboembolic pulmonary disease. J Invasive Cardiol 2019;31(7):E211–9.
50. Kadowaki T, Yano S, Kobayashi K, et al. Pulmonary capillary hemangiomatosis-like foci detected by high resolution computed tomography. Intern Med 2010;49(2):175–8.
51. Resten A, Maitre S, Humbert M, et al. Pulmonary hypertension: CT of the chest in pulmonary venoocclusive disease. AJR American journal of roentgenology 2004;183(1):65–70.
52. Abman SH, Mullen MP, Sleeper LA, et al. Characterisation of paediatric pulmonary hypertensive vascular disease from the PPHNet Registry. Eur Respir J 2022;59(1):2003337.
53. Abman SH, Hansmann G, Archer SL, et al. Pediatric pulmonary hypertension: guidelines from the american heart association and american thoracic society. Circulation 2015;132(21):2037–99.
54. Latus H, Kuehne T, Beerbaum P, et al. Cardiac MR and CT imaging in children with suspected or confirmed pulmonary hypertension/pulmonary hypertensive vascular disease. Expert consensus statement on the diagnosis and treatment of paediatric pulmonary hypertension. The European Paediatric Pulmonary Vascular Disease Network, endorsed by ISHLT and DGPK. Heart 2016;102(Suppl 2):ii30–5.
55. Ratnayaka K, Kanter JP, Faranesh AZ, et al. Radiation-free CMR diagnostic heart catheterization in children. J Cardiovasc Magn Reson 2016;19(1):65.

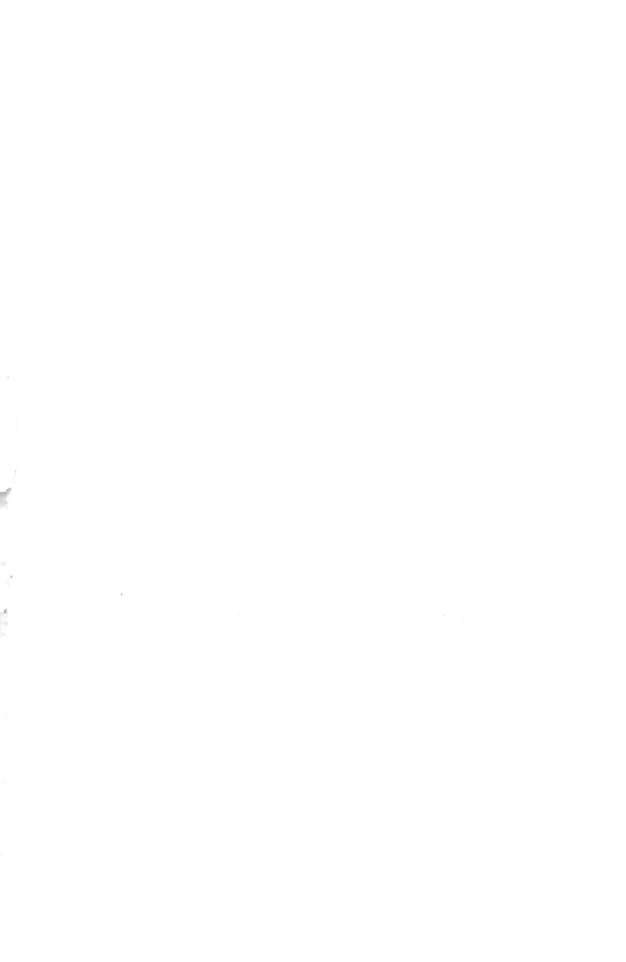